Nonprescription Drugs

Debra A. Lumpe

American Family Health Institute™

Medical Board

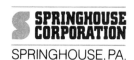

SPRINGHOUSE CORPORATION
SPRINGHOUSE, PA.

Program Director
Stanley Loeb

Clinical Director
Barbara McVan, RN

Art Director
John Hubbard

Editors
Jay Hyams
Susan Cass

**Editorial Services
Supervisor**
David Moreau

Production Manager
Wilbur Davidson

The charter of the American Family Health Institute is to research and produce high-quality publications that enhance the health of individuals and their families. Essential to health are physical, emotional, and social well-being, not just the absence of illness or infirmity. The Institute's Medical Board has produced the *Health and Fitness* books to share up-to-date and authoritative information that can give readers greater personal control over their health maintenance.

Library of Congress Cataloging-in-
Publication Data
Lumpe, Debra A., 1956-
    Nonprescription drugs.
    (Health and fitness series)
    Includes index.
    1. Drugs, Nonprescription. I. Brunner,
Lillian Sholtis.   II. American Family Health
Institute. Medical Board. III. Title. IV. Series.
[DNLM: 1. Drugs, Non-Prescription—popular
works.   QV 772 L958n]
RM671.A1L86   1986   615'.1   85-30275
ISBN 0-87434-025-X

The procedures and explanations given in this publication are based on research and consultation with medical and nursing authorities. To the best of our knowledge, these procedures and explanations reflect currently accepted medical practice; nevertheless, they can't be considered absolute and universal recommendations. For individual application, treatment suggestions must be considered in light of the individual's health, subject to a doctor's specific recommendations. The authors and the publisher disclaim responsibility for any adverse effects resulting directly or indirectly from the suggested procedures, from any undetected errors, or from the reader's misunderstanding of the text.

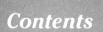

Contents

Nonprescription Drugs

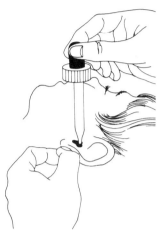

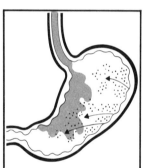

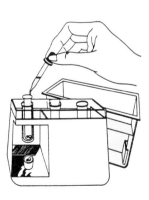

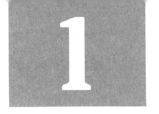

Over-the-counter drugs

Suzy woke up with a headache—again. It was the third time that week she had that heavy, pressing feeling on the left side of her head and face.

"It's probably a sinus headache," Suzy thought. "The weather has changed every day this week." Today she decided she would skip her usual aspirin and stop at the drugstore on the way to work to find something a little stronger to ease the pain. If that didn't work, she would have to ask her friends about finding a doctor. Suzy has lived in the city only a few months and doesn't have a family doctor.

Nonprescription drugs and self-medication

Suzy is not alone in her approach to treating her symptoms. These days few people can afford the time or the money to run to the doctor—if they have one—for every sniffle or headache. Besides, there's no reason to in most cases. Fortunately, nonprescription drugs, also called over-the-counter or OTC products, are readily available in corner drugstores, chain drugstores, supermarkets, and discount houses. They're quick and easy to buy and relatively inexpensive, too. And often they can do the job.

In 1984, Americans spent about $10 billion for a dazzling array of some 300,000 different OTC products. Advertising on television and in newspapers and magazines reminds us which product we can use when we can't sleep, have a sunburn, hemorrhoids, bad breath, or tension headaches. Even douching for "feminine hygiene" is no longer a taboo subject for TV commercials.

Prescription drugs, which must be ordered by a doctor or dentist, are expected to cure an illness. They're usually too strong or addictive to be sold OTC. What nonprescription drugs do is alleviate your symptoms—the stuffy nose, rash from poison ivy, upset stomach. For that reason, there's nothing wrong with self-treatment and self-medication, provided you follow package directions and see a doctor if your symptoms persist for more than a week.

The keys to treating yourself with nonprescription drugs are common sense and moderation. The body has its own mechanisms for warding off germs and fighting infections, so it's best not to rush into self-medication or take too many different products over too long a period of time. You don't want to gum up the works. That way, you'll also be more attuned to your body when you're really sick.

The 1980s has been called America's most health-conscious decade. People everywhere are taking a greater interest in their health. We seek information about the foods we eat and the drugs we take. We're sophisticated enough to take responsibility for our own health care. We can question our doctors about what they're prescribing. And we can find out how nonprescription drugs work in order to treat ourselves.

The FDA review of nonprescription drugs

Foreseeing that trend, the United States Food and Drug Administration (FDA), responsible for overseeing claims made by manufacturers for prescription drugs, decided to review all nonprescription drugs to determine whether they were safe and effective. The FDA, an agency of the Public Health Service, began the review in 1972. It divided all nonprescription drugs into 17 different classes. The medically active ingredients in each class were then examined by an advisory review panel comprised of medical and scientific experts.

The FDA review was precipitated by an amendment to the Food, Drug, and Cosmetic Act, passed by Congress in 1962. Until then, manufacturers could make claims about their nonprescription drugs that may not necessarily have been true. That's because their products didn't have to undergo the same rigorous testing and screening that prescription drugs do.

Each panel's recommendations became and are becoming the basis for new government regulations controlling the manufacture of nonprescription drugs. The FDA expects to finish its review in the late 1980s. Once the process is complete, all drugs sold OTC will be as safe and effective as the regulations can make them. New products will have to meet the more stringent requirements.

Choosing the right product

This book will help you make a decision the next time you're in a drugstore facing a row of different brands and types of medication for one problem and are won-

Approved or not approved

The FDA advisory review panel's assessment of active ingredients in all nonprescription drugs continues. For that reason, you may find some medications on the shelf with ingredients the FDA has not found safe, effective, or either. It's up to you to decide whether to use such products. As with any OTC medication, choose what you think will work best in its simplest form and take the smallest recommended dose.

dering, "Which one is the best for me?" The book will also help you read labels, determine side effects, and guard against harmful drug interactions. In the end, you'll be a wiser and better consumer.

Medicine cabinet basics

Some of this book's chapters cover what are referred to as "medicine cabinet basics." These are products you'll probably want to keep on hand in your home to cover many—if not most—common health problems and emergencies. Besides the pain and fever relievers, these products include the following:

Caution
If you're on a prescription drug, be careful not to use a nonprescription drug that might interfere with or increase the effect of that drug. To be sure, check with your doctor or pharmacist.

- antacids, for when you've had too much to eat or drink and have that "acid indigestion" feeling

- antidiarrheal medications and laxatives, to help regulate your bowels

- products to stop nausea and vomiting

- antihistamines and decongestants, for colds and allergies

- cough relievers, to stop the tickle in your throat

- anti-itch products and antiseptics, to stop itches and treat skin irritations

- skin products, to treat acne, athlete's foot, sunburn, insect stings, and other common skin problems.

Special needs

You'll also find chapters on "special needs"—products you wouldn't normally find in your medicine cabinet. Some of these products are used to treat symptoms of a specific health problem that occurs infrequently and usually doesn't require a doctor's attention, such as hemorrhoids or dandruff. Some of these products are diagnostic tools, tests you can perform yourself to learn certain information about your body. Among the other topics covered are:

- controlling your weight

- what you need to know about contraceptives

- care for your eyes and ears

- mouth care

- what to do about sore throats

- sleep aids and stimulants

- products of special interest to women.

Brand names

This book doesn't make recommendations for or against any specific product. Commonly known brand names—or manufacturer's trade names—are mentioned solely for reference and example. It would be impossible to include all 300,000 products—and new ones are being manufactured every day. The FDA has also recently switched many drugs from a prescription to a nonprescription status. This means you have an even greater number of products to choose from. The agency makes the change when it decides a product has little or no possibility of being harmful when used as directed.

Generic names

The generic name is the drug's chemical name, and the chemicals used in many brand name medicines are available in generic form. For example, Tylenol, Datril, Liquiprin, and Tempra are brand names for the generic drug acetaminophen.

Your doctor's advice

The important thing to remember, however, is never hesitate to ask your doctor for advice. In many cases, he or she may be willing to recommend a product over the telephone at no charge. Or he or she may realize that the symptoms you describe point to a more serious illness than you imagined.

Consult your pharmacist

Pharmacists in drugstores are usually more than willing to answer questions about what a certain drug does, how it should be used, and sometimes even which product they prefer. They'll also know about possible interactions with prescription drugs. If the pharmacist is busy, you may want to make an appointment to see him or her later. Sometimes an assistant will be appointed to answer questions. Either way, their advice is not only professional, it's free.

Better yet, use the same pharmacist for all your drug needs. He or she should keep records of all the prescription medications you're taking. That way, the pharmacist can tell at a glance whether a nonprescription drug will interact negatively. Find a pharmacist who keeps good records. This is especially important if you have more than one doctor, none of whom knows what the other is prescribing.

Active and inactive ingredients

It's important to get to know the active ingredients of the medications you're taking. Most drugs contain both active and inactive ingredients. Active ingredients are those chemicals or compounds that are therapeutic—that is, they alleviate your symptoms. Inactive ingredients are nontherapeutic and include

(text continued on page 10)

What to keep in your medicine cabinet

You'll want to keep your medicine cabinet well stocked with OTC products to deal with common health problems and emergencies. Arrange the products on the cabinet's shelves with dangerous products on the top shelf—out of the reach of children.

Your medicine cabinet should contain a selection of bandages, adhesive dressings, and tape, along with cotton, gauze, and cotton-tipped swabs. These items can go on the bottom shelf along with your toothpaste.

Ammonia inhalants, a thermometer, scissors, tweezers, and pins are also important. Keep them in the door, or in a space away from small children.

Among the OTC products you'll want to have on hand are aspirin or

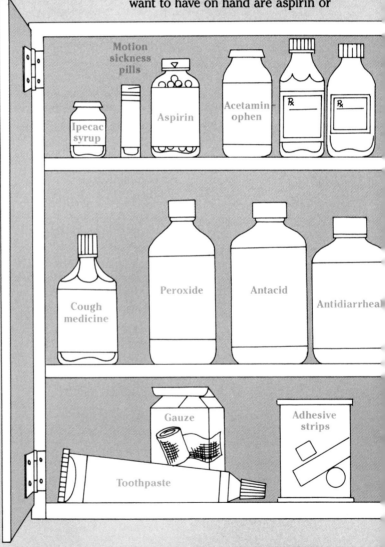

acetaminophen and children's aspirin if there are children in your family; antacid tablets; travel-sickness tablets; ipecac syrup; Kaopectate; calamine lotion, antibacterial cream, or steroid cream; a liquid antiseptic such as hydrogen peroxide; Milk of Magnesia; and cough medicines. All these items belong on the upper shelves, out of reach.

Check your medicine cabinet's contents periodically (at least once a year), and throw out any medicines that have become outdated. Dispose of such products in the toilet, rinse the container, and throw it out—never reuse empty medicine containers. Put the phone number of the nearest poison control center inside the door of the medicine cabinet—and near every phone in your home.

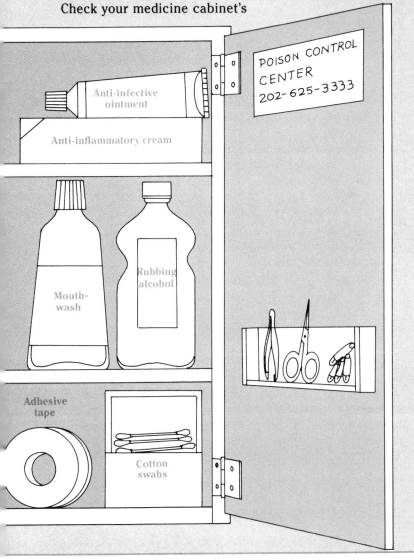

POISON CONTROL CENTER 202-625-3333

Anti-infective ointment

Anti-inflammatory cream

Mouth-wash

Rubbing alcohol

Adhesive tape

Cotton swabs

the coloring, preservatives, or fillers that hold the medication together and give it a shape.

You can compare the active ingredients in two different products. If they're the same, buy the cheaper one. Sometimes it's the store or supermarket brand. It's not recommended that you take any that list more than two active ingredients. These so-called combination products may increase possible negative side effects or drug reactions while providing no greater therapeutic benefit. Some nonprescription drugs, when taken in too large a dose or over an extended period of time, may become harmful or even addictive. That's because they *are* drugs and can affect your body in many ways. It's almost impossible to avoid any and all side effects.

Is more better?
Read labels carefully for active ingredients. The Food and Drug Administration recommends that you not take any drug with more than two active ingredients. This product contains two active ingredients: phenylpropanolamine hydrochloride and dextromethorphan hydrobromide. While giving the active ingredients, this label also tells you how much of each ingredient is contained in a teaspoonful.

Special considerations

Finally, special care should always be taken when you want to use any OTC drugs if you:

• are already taking prescription drugs

• have a chronic disease like diabetes

• intend to give the drug to a child or elderly person

• are pregnant or breast-feeding.

Sodium and high blood pressure

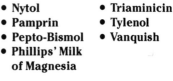

Many people liberally add salt to food often from habit. But for someone with hypertension, this commonly used seasoning is dangerous. Here's why.

Nearly half of salt is comprised of sodium, a mineral that causes fluid retention. Retained fluids can increase blood volume, which in turn boosts blood pressure and puts added pressure on blood vessels.

For anyone on a restricted salt diet, reading labels is essential for selecting sodium-free drugs. (Don't look just for sodium; look for sodium chloride, too.) These products, for example, are sodium-free:

• Bayer
• Bufferin
• CoTylenol
• Comtrex
• Contac
• Coricidin
• Ecotrin
• Excedrin
• Midol
• Nytol
• Pamprin
• Pepto-Bismol
• Phillips' Milk of Magnesia
• Robitussin-DM
• Sine-Aid
• Sine-Off
• Sominex
• Sudafed
• Triaminic Cold Syrup
• Triaminic Expectorant
• Triaminicin
• Tylenol
• Vanquish

2

How to read a label

uzy's head still felt heavy, so she decided to stop in the drugstore on the way to work. She was amazed at how many different products there were. Many boxes claimed to cure not only her sinus headache, but symptoms she didn't even have: runny nose, itchy eyes, cough, and tickle in the throat. She picked up one sinus medication and read that it would help her headache. But it also warned that it might cause drowsiness. "I don't want to fall asleep at work," Suzy thought. "Not with all those reports to do." She kept looking and found a "new, no drowsiness formula" of the same product and carried it to the checkout counter.

What to look for on the label

Pick up a package of the most common OTC medication—aspirin. For example's sake, let's choose Anacin. Aspirin is recommended for a host of symptoms, from headaches and backaches to colds, fevers, and flu. From the package, you see that each bottle contains 100 tablets. Each tablet has two active ingredients: 400 mg aspirin and 32 mg caffeine, about the same amount in one-quarter cup of coffee.

Not all aspirin products contain caffeine. If you're trying to avoid the substance because you already drink enough coffee or soft drinks, or don't want to run the risk of being kept awake, pick a brand with no caffeine. For example, neither Bayer Aspirin nor Bufferin has caffeine.

Reading labels is important, so don't neglect this step. However, many labels are enticements to buy and don't offer much information. Too often the print is small and the words long and technical. Don't be put off by these words. "Acetaminophen" is the active ingredient in Tylenol, just as "aspirin" (acetylsalicylic acid) is in Anacin.

The FDA's evaluation and review of all OTC drugs will soon provide standards for labeling that will include safety and effectiveness. Each product is already required by law to carry on its label a list of the active ingredients and their amounts. If, by chance, a product doesn't list the ingredients, don't buy it. It may be left over on the shelf from before the labeling law.

Caffeine in
over-the-counter drugs
Obvious sources of caffeine
are coffee, tea, and cola;
but caffeine is also in other
foods, beverages, and some
over-the-counter drugs. If
you're trying to avoid caf-
feine, read the label before
buying an over-the-counter
product. Here are some of
the over-the-counter drugs
that contain caffeine.

- **Anacin**
- **Aqua-Ban**
- **Bromo-Seltzer**
- **Caffedrine**
- **Coryban-D**
- **Dexatrim**
- **Dietac**
- **Dristan**
- **Excedrin**
- **Midol**
- **No Doz**
- **Prolamine**
- **Triaminicin**
- **Vanquish**
- **Vivarin**

Some medications can spoil over time. Others lose their potency and become less stable if exposed to humidity, heat, or sunlight. Check the expiration date on each package and don't use the product past the recommended date. If you're buying a large number of tablets, figure out whether you'll have the opportunity to use them all before the expiration date.

The FDA requires each package and product to be labeled with very specific information. For example, a bottle of Extra-Strength Tylenol (acetaminophen) capsules will tell you the following:

1. "Indications: For the temporary relief of minor aches, pains, headaches, and fever." "Indications" means for what symptoms the product is recommended.

2. "Usual Dosage: Adults: Two capsules three or four times daily. No more than a total of eight capsules in any 24-hour period." Notice dosage for children has been omitted. Find another product that includes dosage information for children if you need to give a child an adult drug. Sometimes directions will appear in place of "usual dosage," with the dosage following.

3. "Severe or recurrent pain or high or continued fever may be indicative of serious illness. Under these conditions, consult a physician." This warning is clear enough.

4. "Exp. date 3/87." The drug may not be as potent after this date; it's wisest to throw out what's left and buy some more.

5. "Control number PB4874." This number corresponds with the manufacturer's record of where it was made, what batch, and other information necessary in case that lot must be recalled for any reason.

6. "Extra-Strength Tylenol® acetaminophen capsules contain no aspirin and are unlikely to cause a reaction in those who are allergic to aspirin."

7. "WARNING: Keep this and all medications out of the reach of children. As with any drug, if you are pregnant or nursing a baby, seek the advice of a health professional before using this product. In the case of accidental overdosage, contact a physician or poison control center immediately."

8. "50 capsules—500 mg each." The amount is important because a standard adult unit dose is 325 mg. Taking two extra-strength capsules is not the same as taking two standard tablets.

9. "McNeilab, Inc. Fort Washington, PA 19034 USA." This is the name and location of the manufacturer.

Label information

Read the labels on the OTC products you buy. Along with essential information about how to use the product, you'll find other important information, including:

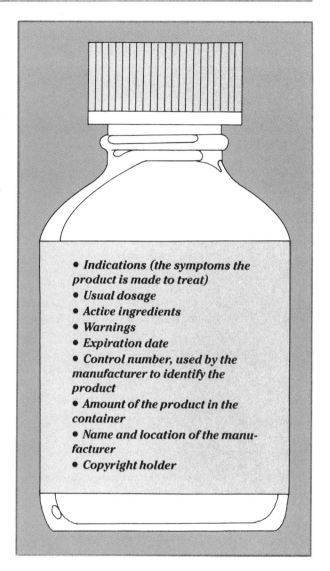

- **Indications (the symptoms the product is made to treat)**
- **Usual dosage**
- **Active ingredients**
- **Warnings**
- **Expiration date**
- **Control number, used by the manufacturer to identify the product**
- **Amount of the product in the container**
- **Name and location of the manufacturer**
- **Copyright holder**

Childproof caps

If you have children or if children frequently visit your home, you should use childproof caps. These are available on the containers of many OTC products as well as on the containers of many household products. Although they make opening the product a little harder, they're well worth the bother—they save children's lives.

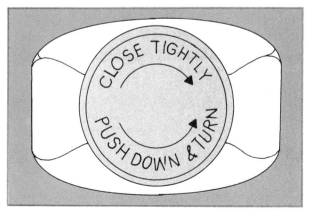

10. "Package not child-resistant." This is important if you have a child in the house.

11. "© McN '84." Copyright holder.

Other information you may find on labels includes the distributor, if different from the manufacturer, and other advice, such as "Store at room temperature," "Take with food or milk if occasional and mild heartburn, upset stomach, or stomach pain occurs with use," or "The smallest effective dose should be used."

Has the package been tampered with?

Examine each package you buy to make sure it hasn't been tampered with. Check the wrappings and seals to see whether they've been broken. All products are now required by the FDA to be "tamper-proof," following the Tylenol capsule scare. In 1982, seven people in the Chicago area died after ingesting what they believed were Tylenol capsules. Authorities believe that capsules containing a poisonous substance were put in the bottles after the bottles left the manufacturing plant and probably while they were sitting on the store's shelf.

Most OTC packages tell you what to look for to determine whether the product has been tampered with, such as "Do not use if red neck wrap or foil inner seal is broken," or "Do not buy if sticker or carton flaps have been broken."

Patient package insert

Sometimes the product will include a sheet of information and instructions inside the package. This is called a "PPI," or patient package insert. Read this carefully, because it will usually tell you more than what's on the package or the label. Drug tablets or capsules will usually also be labeled. Some are imprinted with the name of the drug or manufacturer and the amount of the active ingredient.

Precautions

Remember that any drug's listed indications and dosages are intended for an average person's use. No two people are alike. Follow the directions on the labels or packaging. Don't exceed the recommended dose: more of the drug does not ensure faster or better relief of symptoms and is likely to cause harm. Check with your doctor if symptoms don't clear up in the amount of time listed in the directions, or if you are taking prescription drugs. Many OTC products can interfere with prescription drugs.

Tamper-proof packaging

Tamper-proof packaging has several forms. A tamper-proof box may be sealed with special tape or with a seal; don't buy the product if the box's seal or tape is broken. Five types of tamper-proof packages are illustrated here:

• Plastic seals surrounding bottle or container caps

• Paper or plastic stickers placed over box top openings

• Inner foil seals

• Cellophane wrappers for boxes

• Adhesive closures for box tops and bottoms.

Other kinds of tamper-proof packaging include:

• Metal canisters with pull-top metal lids

• "Kapseals": two-part capsules that can't be opened

• Blister packs: molded plastic over pills that protects the pills and also alerts you to any tampering

• Bottle closures that indicate whether or not the bottle has been opened; if opened, the message "opened" is locked into place.

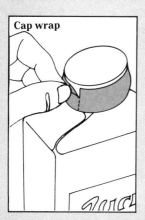

Cap wrap

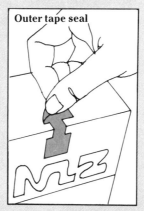

Outer tape seal

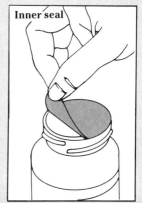

Inner seal

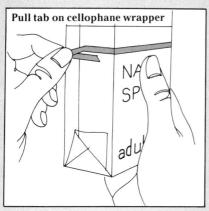

Pull tab on cellophane wrapper

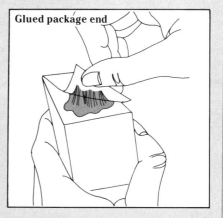

Glued package end

3

Antacids

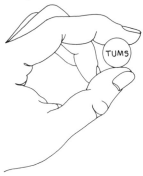

TUMS

Tablets and capsules are usually imprinted with the name of the drug. Sometimes a lot number or milligram amount appears, too.

Antacids and calcium
Antacids are also now being touted as a good source of calcium. Calcium is essential in preventing osteoporosis, a fragile bone condition that can plague older people.

The National Institutes of Health recommend a daily calcium and Vitamin D supplement for women to help prevent osteoporosis. However, according to some doctors, any generic brand of calcium carbonate is as good as a name brand. Make sure you check how much of the ingredient is in each tablet; it can range from 47 mg (Calcium Gluconate, Lilly) to 600 mg (Caltrate 600, Lederle).

Antacids are usually taken for indigestion, which is a catchall for many different symptoms. These symptoms can include heartburn, cramps, gas pains, or a bloated feeling from eating too much food. There are about 575 different antacid products you can buy in many forms—tablets, lozenges, liquids, gels, capsules, chewing gum, and powders.

There are many causes of indigestion. It's important to recognize which one you might be experiencing. There's a difference between feeling mildly uncomfortable after eating a too-spicy meal and the feeling that signals a heart attack, a common—and important—cause of symptoms of indigestion in middle-aged men. Sometimes indigestion may be a side effect of prescription drugs such as antibiotics.

You should call your doctor for indigestion if certain conditions are present. These include one severe attack, especially if you also feel weak, out-of-breath, and are sweating; if you vomit blood; or if your indigestion repeats itself, even if only a few times a month over several months. Don't try to treat yourself if any of these three conditions is present or persists because it may mean you have a serious medical problem that a doctor should know about right away.

Acid indigestion is a symptom of too much stomach acid, or hyperacidity. Antacids neutralize hydrochloric acid, which is secreted by the glands lining the stomach wall. Hydrochloric acid is produced to help digest food, but sometimes too much is produced or is produced when no food is present.

What antacids can and can't do
The FDA advisory review panel on OTC antacid drugs made a clear finding about what manufacturers can claim their products can do. The agency found that antacids can relieve heartburn, sour stomach, acid indigestion, and an upset stomach related to those symptoms, but that's it. Thus, the only symptoms you should try to treat yourself are those caused by an excess of such stomach acid. These symptoms include a burning feeling in your stomach, upper abdomen, and even the throat. Companies that claim otherwise about their products can't prove it scientifically. The

Antacids and digestion

Some people take antacids when they've eaten too much, yet an antacid is made to counter the digestive acid in your stomach, and you need the acid when you've overeaten.

FDA found false or misleading claims made by products to relieve any of the following: "gas," "upper abdominal pressure," "full feeling," "nausea," "excessive eructations [belching]," "sour breath," "nervous and emotional disturbances," "excessive smoking," "food intolerance," "consumption of alcoholic beverages," "nervous-tension headaches," "cold symptoms," or "morning sickness of pregnancy."

Ingredients in antacids

There are four ingredients in antacids to look for: sodium bicarbonate, calcium carbonate, aluminum compounds, and magnesium compounds. Some antacids contain one of the ingredients, but most contain at least two. The FDA allows up to four to be combined.

Unlike other active ingredients in nonprescription drugs, those in antacids are considered safer in that the only way a person can harm himself is by taking too much over a long period of time. In fact, peptic ulcers are sometimes treated with large doses of antacids. You should be careful, however, if you're also taking a prescription drug containing tetracycline. Antacids can negate the drug's effects. Wait at least three hours after taking tetracycline before you use an antacid.

Acid indigestion

That "acid indigestion feeling" is caused by the production of too much hydrochloric acid, which is secreted by glands that line the stomach wall (see arrows). Antacids neutralize this hydrochloric acid, relieving the burning feeling in your stomach, upper abdomen, or throat.

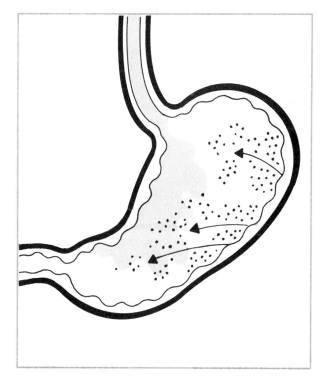

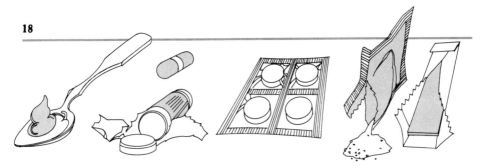

The choice is yours

Antacids are sold in many different forms, including liquids, capsules, tablets, lozenges, powder in packets, and chewing gum. Choose the form you prefer; just be sure to look for these ingredients: sodium bicarbonate, calcium carbonate, aluminum compounds, and magnesium compounds. Some will have only one, others a combination of two or more. Choose a product that doesn't upset your bowel function.

Always dissolve first

Effervescent tablets such as Alka-Seltzer contain aspirin, which helps relieve pain. These tablets should always be dissolved in water before you swallow them, because they have a high bicarbonate content that can cause gastric irritation. If you're taking them for an upset stomach, swallowing them undissolved could cause you more pain.

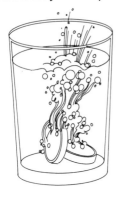

The FDA has also approved other active ingredients for antacids:

- bismuth compounds
- citrates
- glycine
- dried milk solids
- phosphate compounds
- potassium compounds
- silicates
- tartrate compounds.

Several familiar antacids containing safe and effective ingredients include Tums, Rolaids, Di-Gel tablets, Mylanta, Gelusil, WinGel, Riopan, and Bromo Seltzer. Plain old baking soda (sodium bicarbonate) is also effective. Most people apparently choose an antacid by its taste and effect on their bowels.

Guidelines for treating yourself with antacids

- Don't use an antacid regularly for more than a few weeks without your doctor's knowledge and advice.

- Restrict use of sodium bicarbonate or calcium carbonate antacids. Instead, choose products that contain ingredients like aluminum and magnesium.

- Watch the sodium content of antacids. Two tablets of Alka-Seltzer contain more than 1,000 mg of sodium. Any dose more than 9 mg sodium is considered too high if you're on a low-salt or sodium-restricted diet.

- Antacids in liquid or suspension form seem to work best. Insoluble particles floating in a liquid are in suspension. Examples of suspension antacids include Phillips' Milk of Magnesia and Maalox.

- Chew or suck antacid tablets thoroughly. The more they're dissolved, the more effective they'll be. There's no guarantee they'll be completely dissolved in the stomach if you swallow them.

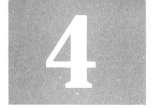

Antidiarrheals and laxatives

The bowel movement can be a subject of great concern to some people. Their concern is heightened by misunderstanding. Nowhere is it inscribed that unless you have a daily bowel movement, you're constipated. Yet there are more than 700 laxative products available in drugstores, on which Americans annually spend an estimated $350 million at last count.

Regularity

Before buying and using a laxative, you should first understand your body and its daily rhythms. If you don't already know what's "regular" for you—and that means regular intervals, not daily—keep a record for a couple of weeks. Chart the dates and times you have bowel movements. For some people, regular may be three times a day; for others, every three days. What's important is not to worry needlessly, because stress can also be a cause of constipation and diarrhea.

Once you know what's normal for you, you can recognize when you have a problem you can treat yourself. For example, one day of diarrhea might just mean you've eaten something that didn't agree with you. If it persists, however, you may have an intestinal virus that warrants stronger treatment if not a visit to the doctor. Often diarrhea is accompanied by nausea or an upset stomach.

Sometimes what you eat speeds up the process or slows it down. Besides stress, traveling can cause constipation. Taking a laxative should never be considered "natural," but in these cases, a mild laxative taken for a couple of days will produce no harmful effects. But be careful when you feel prolonged or severe abdominal pain. Such pain is almost never associated with constipation and never calls for laxatives. Instead, the pain may be caused by appendicitis or another acute illness.

Constipation can also be linked to childhood toilet-training habits, suppression of the urge to defecate, crowded living conditions, or poor exercise or eating habits. In a few cases, constipation may be the result of cancer or a digestive disease like diverticulosis. However, in these instances a definite change in either frequency of bowel movements or their color and consistency is noticeable. Such instances are relatively rare, however, and are usually found in older people. If you've had a constipation problem for a number of years, then a disease is probably not the cause.

Types of laxatives

If, after changing your diet to include more liquids and roughage, you still want to use a laxative, there are several different types to choose from.

The first are called bulk-forming laxatives, which means they work by increasing the bulk and water content of the stool. Others include stimulant laxatives, which promote the motion of the bowel; saline laxatives, which draw water into the bowel; hyperosmotic laxatives, which increase the stool's water content; stool-softener laxatives; and lubricant laxatives, which help to ease out the stool.

The FDA advisory panel found the only accurate claim that these products can make is "laxative [for the] short-term relief of constipation." No reference can be made to either promoting good health or changing "irregularity."

Besides bran, bulk laxatives containing the active ingredient psyllium, such as Metamucil and Effersyllium, are recommended. Always be sure to drink a glass of water with a bulk laxative to help make it work. If you're taking aspirin or prescription drugs such as digitalis or nitrofurantoin, however, don't take a bulk laxative, because it prevents absorption of these drugs.

The other categories of laxatives should all be used with caution. Many are hard on the body, robbing it of essential nutrients. Hyperosmotic laxatives should be used only in the suppository form. A lubricant laxative such as mineral oil is slow-acting and softens fecal matter, but it also interferes with digestion and absorption of some nutrients. Saline laxatives such as the magnesium, phosphate, and tartar salts are recommended. Milk of Magnesia is one example.

As with other OTC drugs, check the ingredients. No more than two active ingredients should be combined in one medication. Don't overuse or become dependent on laxatives to keep you regular. If you have hemorrhoids or other anorectal irritation, avoid using laxatives. Instead, try exercise, more roughage in your diet, and try to reduce stress. Save the laxatives for mild cases of constipation, such as when you travel.

Is a laxative the answer?

Before rushing out to buy another laxative, take a minute to review your eating habits. Is your diet adequate in grains and cereals, fruits and vegetables, and daily liquids? High-protein diets usually cause constipation. Even exercise can complicate your bowel's habits if your intake of fluids is too low. Remember, also, that some medications cause constipation, and you may have recently taken one.

Diarrhea

Besides being embarrassing and physically incapaci-tating, diarrhea is often accompanied by headaches, nausea, chills, a fever, and cramps. If you have diarrhea for more than two days, if it's accompanied by a fever, or if the stools are black or bloody, see a doctor. Children younger than 3 with diarrhea should also see a doctor.

Most OTC remedies for diarrhea do no more than relieve symptoms for the mildest cases. Such diarrhea can be caused by bad food or drink, an intestinal virus, or other illnesses. In fact, diarrhea can be linked to as many as 50 different conditions.

The first thing to do if you have a mild case of diarrhea is to cut out all solid foods and begin a clear liquid diet. That's because diarrhea is really excess water that remains in your intestine during digestion instead of being absorbed by the body. You need to replace this water so you don't become dehydrated. Also, get plenty of rest and avoid tobacco, caffeine, and alcohol. If your diarrhea is a little more severe, take an absorb-ent like Kaopectate. This is a combination of kaolin, a claylike substance, and pectin, a plant extract. It works by binding to the excess water. Other remedies include ingredients such as bismuth subsalicylate, or Pepto-Bismol, and polycarbophil, an indigestible synthetic resin. The latter is the only OTC antidiarrheal recom-mended by the FDA for use in children.

Interestingly, the FDA panel found only two active ingredients both safe and effective for the treatment of mild diarrhea. Besides polycarbophil, mentioned above, opium powder, tincture of opium, and pare-goric were found to be the safest and most effective of all antidiarrheal remedies. The FDA recommended that the opium be combined with another active ingre-dient to prevent any addiction.

How diarrhea occurs

Diarrhea may result from excessive contractions of muscles in the digestive tract. Normally, a series of these wavelike muscle con-tractions—called peristalsis—forces food through the digestive tract. But if peri-stalsis occurs too quickly, the large intestine doesn't absorb as much fluid as it should from food. This leads to diarrhea.

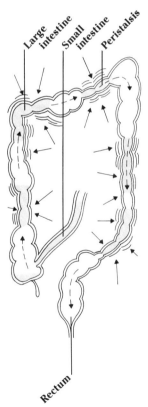

5 Antihistamines and decongestants

Symptoms of the common cold include a runny, stuffy, and congested nose, sore throat, hoarseness, coughs both with and without a congested chest, headache, fever, and muscular aches. There's the adage that modern science has yet to come up with a cure for the common cold. This remains true.

What cold-relief products can do

No antihistamine or decongestant will do anything for you but alleviate the cold's symptoms while the cold runs its course. What your mother always told you is still true: get plenty of bed rest, humidify the air, drink plenty of fluids, and eat a well-balanced diet.

Colds are infections that attack the membrane lining the upper respiratory tract, which is made up of the nose, throat, sinuses, and bronchial passages. But the inherent problem in treating the common cold is that not all colds are the same. In fact, more than 125 different viruses can cause a cold. About 60 head straight for the lining of your nose. Most colds run their own course in one to two weeks.

There are more than 200 different brand-name products in drugstores that will relieve cold symptoms. They contain either an antihistamine, decongestant, a combination of the two, or a combination with an analgesic, or pain reliever. The antihistamine is

How to use nose drops

- *Lie down on your back on a bed or couch with your head hanging slightly over the edge.*
- *Draw medication into the nose dropper.*
- *Insert the dropper about 3/8 inch into a nostril. Make sure the dropper doesn't touch the sides of the nostril.*
- *Release the prescribed number of drops.*

- *Keep your head tilted back for at least five minutes and breathe out of your mouth.*
- *Sit upright and spit out any liquid that has drained into your mouth.*

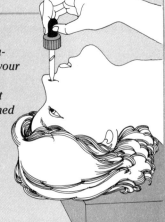

usually chlorpheniramine, as in Chlor-Trimeton.

Decongestants work by shrinking swollen membranes and small blood vessels in the lining of the nose. Antihistamines work by blocking allergic reactions caused by histamines, substances found in the body. They also help to dry mucus.

Antihistamines have very little effect—if any—on helping you get over your stuffy nose. For this reason most major cold pills contain a combination of decongestant and antihistamine. These products include Afrin, Neo-Synephrine, Dristan, Contac, and Sinarest. It's wiser to buy antihistamines and decongestants separately, though, and perhaps also get a medication such as nose sprays, drops, or inhalants for those colds that begin with a stuffy, runny nose.

Don't use any medications in the nose for more than three or four days, however, because overuse can give you the same symptoms you started with or clog up the passages even more. Follow directions carefully when you use any product in the nose. You'll probably taste the medication, but don't worry about it.

The best relief for a cold with an accompanying headache, fever, or muscle ache is an analgesic and a decongestant. The combination of an antihistamine and decongestant is usually the best treatment for minor allergies.

Caffeine is a common ingredient in antihistamines. It's added to counteract the drowsiness these products can cause. The average amount is about what you would get from drinking a quarter cup of coffee. If

Caution
Avoid taking oral decongestants if you have high blood pressure, hyperthyroidism, or take certain antidepressant drugs. If you feel agitated and start to suffer from insomnia, you may be taking too much decongestant.

Caution
Don't use nose drops or nasal sprays for more than three days. Overuse can make your problem worse.

How to use a nasal spray

To get the most benefit out of using a nasal spray or drops, cover and penetrate the area with the solution. To use a nasal spray, stand or sit upright, tilt your head back, insert the nozzle into one nostril, and squeeze the bottle firmly and quickly. Repeat for a total of two to three times, and then do the same in the other nostril. Use in the morning and at night.

you're drowsy a lot of the time, cut back on the antihistamines.

Another common additive in colds products is alcohol, especially in cough syrups and liquid suspensions. It's used primarily to help dissolve the active ingredients. Carefully check the concentration levels of alcohol listed on the package and label. Some products may contain only 1 percent alcohol; others may be as high as 42 percent. Most wines have only a 12 percent alcohol content.

You should avoid products with more than minimal percentages of alcohol if you plan to give the medication to a child, are diabetic, or are taking prescription drugs for depression or anxiety or both.

Asthma

If your ailment is not relieved by antihistamines or decongestants and you have trouble breathing, a persistent cough and a wheeze, you may have asthma, a more serious form of hay fever. If you get these symptoms, see a doctor rather than treat yourself.

However, if you already know you have asthma, you're probably taking drugs called bronchodilators, which relax the muscles of the airway so you can breathe normally. These drugs are extremely powerful. They can make the heart race and pound, raise blood pressure, and cause sleeplessness, nausea, vomiting, and nervousness.

For these reasons, OTC bronchodilators should be used only for "temporary relief of bronchial asthma, and only be bought by those who have already been diagnosed as having asthma." If you don't get relief within 20 minutes to an hour, call your doctor or have someone take you to a hospital emergency room.

The FDA advisory panel has approved active ingredients from two groups of drugs to be used in bronchodilators. They're either sympathomimetics or the theophyllines. Both work by inhibiting enzymes that prevent the passages from being relaxed. The active ingredients include:

• Ephedrine preparations

• Epinephrine preparations

• Methoxyphenamine hydrochloride

• Theophylline preparations.

Brand names for bronchodilators include Asthma-Haler, Bronkaid Mist, and Primatene Mist.

Allergy symptoms

Hay fevers or mild allergies produce symptoms similar to colds, except hay fever lasts longer, never produces a fever, and is accompanied by itchy eyes or nose. Hay fever is treated primarily with antihistamines.

How to use a bronchodilator

Inhaling the medication in a bronchodilator will help you breathe more easily. Here's how to use a bronchodilator.

1

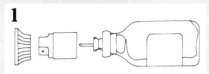

Remove the mouthpiece and cap from the bottle. Then remove the cap from the mouthpiece.

2

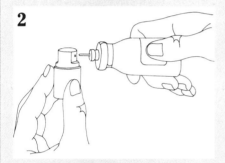

Turn the mouthpiece sideways. On one side of the flattened tip, you'll see a small hole. Fit the metal stem on the bottle into the hole.

3

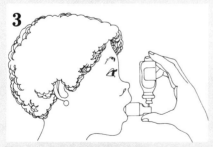

Now exhale. Hold the bronchodilator upside-down, as shown here, and close your lips loosely around the mouthpiece.

4

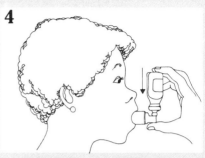

Inhale slowly. As you do, firmly push the bottle against the mouthpiece— one time only—to release one dose of medicine. Continue inhaling until your lungs feel full.

5

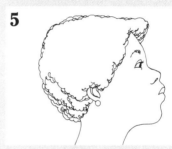

Take the mouthpiece away from your mouth, and hold your breath momentarily.

6

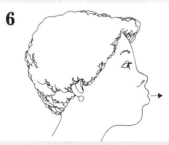

Purse your lips and exhale slowly. If the doctor suggests, repeat the procedure. Important: never overuse your bronchodilator. Follow your doctor's instructions exactly. Finally, rinse the mouthpiece with warm water.

6

Anti-itch products and antiseptics

Medic Alert bracelets
If you have a medical condition that others should know about in case of an emergency—such as a severe allergic reaction to insect stings—wear a Medic Alert bracelet. These bracelets are available from the Medic Alert Foundation International, 2323 Colorado, P.O. Box 1009, Turlock, California 95381; telephone, (800) 344-3226.

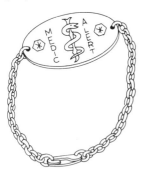

The skin is a fascinating organ. It covers the entire surface of the body, keeping out infection and germs. It's vastly different, depending on what section of the body it's protecting: thin and sensitive over the lips, nose, and ears; thick and armorlike on the soles of the feet.

Sometimes the skin mirrors what is happening systemically in our bodies, such as a rash associated with measles or the acne set in motion by hormonal imbalances. In other cases, the skin reacts to external forces: the sting of a wasp causes swelling and redness; too much sun produces a sunburn.

What you reach for to help your skin problem depends on your symptoms. In this chapter, anti-itch agents and antiseptics are discussed. Antiseptics prevent infection by destroying microorganisms on the skin. Both types of products are usually found in a first-aid kit for insect stings and bites, rashes from poison ivy, poison oak, and poison sumac, and for small wounds such as scrapes and cuts.

Insect bites and stings

Insect bites and stings range from the innocuous but irritating and itchy bump produced by a mosquito to the life-threatening (if you're allergic to the insect's toxin) sting of a wasp. Besides wasps, stinging insects that can cause serious and harmful effects include honeybees and bumblebees, yellow jackets, and hornets.

If you've ever been stung by a bee or a wasp, you'll recall the initial pain, followed by a throbbing feeling, swelling, redness, and an intense itching that hurts even more when you scratch. What your body is reacting to is the poison, or toxin, injected by the offending insect with its sting. This reaction can be made worse if you scratch, because dirt and bacteria can enter the wound.

If stung by a bee, remove the stinger by scraping it out with a fingernail or knife blade. Don't squeeze it out: doing so will only release more venom into the wound. Wash the area carefully with soap and water. Put ice on it to reduce the swelling.

Next, apply an antiseptic. The best choice is isopropyl alcohol, approved by the FDA panel in concentra-

Keeping pests away

Using external insect repellents is a good way to prevent having to use OTC medications for bites and stings. They come in the form of sprays, creams, lotions, sticks, or on towelettes. You should cover all exposed parts of your body, avoiding the eyes, lips, and areas with cuts or sunburn. Read the label to make sure the product won't stain clothes. There are no approved ingredients you can take internally to ward off unwelcome insect attackers.

Insect repellents fall under the jurisdiction of the Environmental Protection Agency (EPA), not the Food and Drug Administration. That's because they contain the insecticide N,N-diethyl-meta-toluamide, also known as deet, as their active ingredient. All insect repellents are labeled with an EPA registration number, followed by an establishment number that's been assigned to a particular manufacturer.

For example, OFF Insect Repellent (Johnson & Johnson) is labeled, "EPA Reg# 4822-10; EPA EST-4288-WI-1." Check for a similar number and for deet. Most will contain varying percentages of this substance. For example, Skeeter Stop 100 (Outdoor Recreation Product) contains 95 percent deet.

Hornet

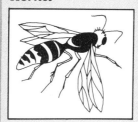

Hornets hang their large, pear-shaped nests from tree limbs. They don't attack unless their nest is threatened.

Yellow jacket

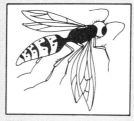

Yellow jackets build their nests in trees, holes in the ground, tree stumps, or walls. They're very aggressive and quick-tempered.

Honeybee

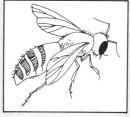

Honeybees have round, smooth abdomens and build nests in hollow trees or in the ground. They can be quite aggressive when defending the area around their nests. They release "alarm odors" that alert other nearby bees to join in the attack on a victim, and this can lead to multiple stings.

Bumblebee

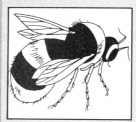

Bumblebees are 2 to 3 times larger than honeybees, have furry, rounded abdomens, and make a noisy buzzing sound. They aren't as aggressive as honeybees and will rarely attack unless a nest, located in the ground, is stepped upon.

tions of 50 percent to 91.3 percent. It's usually called rubbing alcohol. It's inexpensive, very effective, and the least irritating to the skin. In addition, few people are allergic to it. The FDA panel also approved ethyl alcohol, in concentrations of 60 percent to 90 percent, for use as an antiseptic.

Very hot or very cold compresses may stop the itching. A 0.5 percent concentration of hydrocortisone in a cream base may also help. The FDA now allows two preparations from a class of drugs called corticosteroids to be sold: hydrocortisone and hydrocortisone acetate. These two active ingredients in antipruritics used to be available only by prescription.

There are many different kinds of remedies for itchy, painful skin. All work a little differently, but overall

If you're stung

After being stung, most people experience only a localized reaction at the site of the wound. That's because the amount of venom injected by the insect is too small to produce any greater response. About 10 percent of the U.S. population, however, is extremely sensitive to the venom. Allergic symptoms in these cases can include

- nausea
- vomiting
- fainting
- sweating
- fever
- chills
- headache
- muscle soreness
- breathing problems.

In some cases, heart failure, shock, and even death may result. It's important to get immediate emergency attention because with each sting, a person becomes more

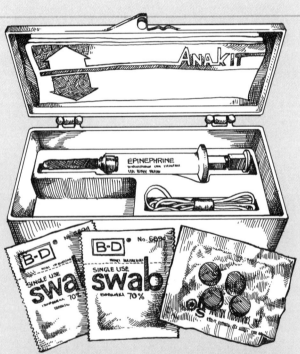

sensitive and may have reactions that get progressively worse. You probably already know if you have severe allergies to bites and stings. If so, carry identification to tell others of this allergy. It's

also not a bad idea to carry your own emergency kit, containing a tourniquet and a preloaded syringe of epinephrine (known as Adrenalin), available from your doctor.

Removing a stinger

Bees have barbed stingers that become firmly anchored in human skin. When the bee tries to free itself—or when the victim brushes it off—the stinger and its attached venom sac break off. Minus this part of its body, the bee flies off and dies; the stinger, embedded in the skin, continues to pump venom into the victim.

If you're stung by a bee, you'll need to remove the bee's stinger before performing any other first aid measures. Don't use tweezers to remove a stinger. Squeezing the stinger will only release more venom into the

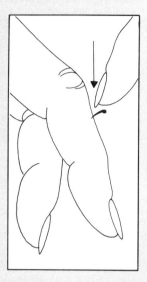

wound. Scrape away the stinger with a fingernail or the edge of a knife blade. Having removed the stinger, wash the wound with soap and water and apply an antiseptic. If available, apply ice to the wound. This will help reduce the swelling.

The pain and irritation can be relieved with the application of a paste made from baking soda and water; however, some doctors recommend the application of meat tenderizer (any brand will do). Make a paste of 1/4 of a teaspoon of meat tenderizer added to about 1 or 2 teaspoons of water.

they're called external analgesics. Because the FDA panel found more than three dozen active ingredients in OTC medications safe and effective, it attempted to classify them pharmacologically, or according to how they work in the body. There are five groups:

- anesthetics
- alcohols
- antihistamines
- salicylates
- corticosteroids.

Examples of products considered external analgesics for pain and itching include D-Caine (Century), Wellcortin (Burroughs Wellcome), Cortaid (Upjohn), and Xylocaine (Astra).

Insects that feed on blood bite. These insects include ticks, chiggers, mosquitoes, fleas, bedbugs, and lice. Of all these, mosquito bites generally respond the best to relief offered by nonprescription medication. The other insects, which tend to attach themselves firmly to our skin in order to maintain a constant blood supply, may require stronger remedies. While OTC drugs may provide temporary relief, you should consult your doctor to identify the insect—and any eggs it may have laid—and recommend stronger treatment. Ticks, for example, should not just be pulled out, because their heads can remain imbedded in the skin.

Poison ivy and contact dermatitis

Besides insect bites and stings, another cause of severe, intense itching is contact with poison ivy, poison oak, or poison sumac. Contact is most likely in the spring. These plants produce an oily resin, an allergen, that causes allergic reactions to the skin by direct or indirect exposure. Indirect exposure can include your dog or cat brushing against your legs after it has run through poison ivy.

Symptoms begin a few hours after contact. In some cases, swollen sores or blisters may appear. The fluid in these blisters isn't contagious. The best treatment remains calamine lotion and very hot or cold compresses. You can also take an analgesic.

If you can't trace your rash to contact with a plant or a bite, you may be allergic to various household items such as glue, detergent, or even the dye in your clothing. One woman reported a rash on her forearms, and after trial and error finally linked it to an inexpensive pair of rubber gloves that had dissolved inside when put in too-hot water. These kinds of rashes are called contact dermatitis.

An allergy may develop

Even if you've never had a bad reaction to poison ivy, oak, or sumac, you may become susceptible. For some people, it takes many years of repeated exposures to develop a sensitivity. Some people never develop the allergy; some are allergic all their lives.

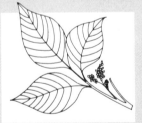

Poison ivy
- Leaves always consist of three glossy leaflets
- Grows as a small plant, a vine, or a shrub
- Grows everywhere in the United States except California and parts of adjacent states

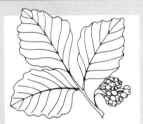

Poison oak
- Leaves always consist of three leaflets
- Grows as a shrub or vine
- Grows in California and parts of adjacent states

Most rashes you'll treat yourself will be found in only one or a few areas of the body. However, if much of the body is covered and the rash is accompanied by severe swelling and you have a fever, you should contact your doctor. In some instances, very severe cases of poison ivy, oak, or sumac or contact dermatitis will also need a doctor's attention.

Your main goals in treating these rashes will be to reduce the urge to scratch and to dry out sores. But be careful: too much medication may cause additional allergic reactions or secondary infections because of over-scrubbing.

Scrapes and cuts

You can also treat scrapes, cuts, and similar small wounds yourself. As with stings and bites, first clean the wound gently with soap and water. Dirt and gravel should be removed by careful scrubbing or with a pair of tweezers. Then use alcohol as an antiseptic. Don't pour it directly into the wound, but swab around it. Cover it with a small bandage to keep out any additional germs. Don't make it airtight.

Besides alcohol, other antiseptics to clean wounds include:

• antibiotics, such as bacitracin. The FDA panel found "that no potential for harm exists when bacitracin is used on small wounds such as small cuts, abrasions, or burns."

• halogens, such as iodine, sold as Betadine (Purdue Frederick).

• quaternary ammonium compounds, such as benzalkonium chloride. These are effective against gram-positive organisms, such as staphylococci, and gram-negative bacteria. Both cause skin infections. OTC medications include Bactine Hydrocortisone Skin Care Cream (Miles).

• hydrogen peroxide, 3 percent solution, is found in many medicine cabinets. When poured over a wound, it froths at the edges and may clean particularly dirty wounds. However, overall it's not a very good antiseptic.

In general, the body's defenses seem quite able to cope with many of the small abrasions we suffer, including skin infections. This is just as well, because the FDA panel found no OTC antibiotic intended for skin infections to be safe or effective.

Caution

If you're cut deeper than ³⁄₈ of an inch, you may need a tetanus shot if you have not had one in 10 years. See a doctor immediately.

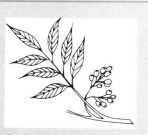

Poison sumac

• *Grows as a woody shrub or small tree from 5 to 25 feet tall*
• *Grows in most of the eastern third of the United States*

7

Contraceptives

Technical names

Nonoxynol-9 and octoxynol 9, active ingredients in OTC vaginal contraceptives, may not be listed by these shortened names. Instead, they may be listed by their chemical compounds. Don't be put off by these technical names—they mean the same thing:

Nonoxynol-9 nonylphenoxypolyethoxyethanol, nonyl phenoxy polyoxyethylene ethanol, polyosyethylenenonylphenol.

Octoxynol 9 p-diisobutylphenenoxypolyethoxyethanol, polyethylene glycol of mono-iso-octyl phenyl ether.

Contraceptives are used to prevent pregnancy. Men can use condoms, a sheath that fits over the erect penis to collect sperm after ejaculation. This sheath is usually made of thin latex rubber, hence its nickname, "rubber." The FDA panel didn't review condoms, because they contain no active ingredients and don't need approval to be sold. However, condoms made of lamb intestines are not as stringently tested for flaws and should be avoided. Pharmacies and drugstores usually carry a variety of condoms.

Vaginal contraceptives

Besides oral contraceptives, which must be prescribed by a doctor, or an IUD, which must be inserted by a doctor and is not recommended for women who have not yet had children, many types of nonprescription vaginal contraceptives are available. There are creams, foams, jellies, suppositories, and sponges. All serve the same purpose: to prevent sperm from entering the uterus and ultimately uniting with a fertile egg. They accomplish this either by forming a barrier over the opening of the cervix or by killing sperm by means of a spermicide. Sperm cells are usually killed within seconds after contact with a spermicide.

The FDA panel approved only two spermicidal active ingredients as safe and effective: nonoxynol-9 and octoxynol 9, both almost identical in chemical structure. Most vaginal OTC contraceptives sold in the U.S. contain either one or the other of these ingredients. No combination products were approved.

Conception

Conception occurs when a sperm reaches a fertile egg. Each ejaculation can release millions of sperm, which move up through the cervix to fertilize the egg in the uterus.

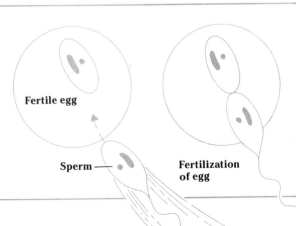

Fertile egg

Sperm

Fertilization of egg

Inactive ingredients

You may wonder about all the other ingredients listed on the package. Most give the foam, jelly, cream, or suppository its shape, smell, and consistency. These are called inactive ingredients, and they're numerous. Included are:

- *acacia*
- *alcohol*
- *benzethonium chloride*
- *boric acid*
- *butylparaben*
- *deionized water*
- *glycerin*
- *hydroxyethylcellulose*
- *methylbenzethonium chloride*
- *methylparaben*
- *methyl polysiloxane*
- *perfume*
- *preservatives*
- *propylparaben*
- *purified water*
- *sodium borate*
- *starch*
- *stearic acid*
- *tragacanth.*

Fertilized egg

No major side effects have been reported with the use of vaginal contraceptives. However, the FDA panel found few studies that evaluated the safety of spermicidal ingredients. As a result, the panel called for new guidelines with which to measure vaginal contraceptives. They:

- must act quickly, either to kill all sperm on contact or render them incapable of fertilization

- must be free of long-term toxicity to the mother and her offspring

- must not be harmful to a recently conceived fetus

- must not be systemically toxic to the woman or irritating either to her vagina or her mate's penis.

Not all products work the same, however, and their effectiveness can vary. Much depends on how they're used, and whether women follow the directions correctly. For example, foams must be used right before intercourse and then reapplied if intercourse is repeated. Suppositories, on the other hand, take approximately 15 minutes to melt and may not be as effective in providing protection before then.

Women sometimes make mistakes in administering contraceptives. Some don't push in the cream far enough; others may not like to touch their vaginas, making use of such products risky. Some women believe that douching after intercourse is a reliable means of contraception. Unfortunately, the price of learning this is not the case is usually unwanted pregnancy. According to the FDA panel, douching is not effective because it can't be done quickly enough to kill sperm, which can reach the uterus within minutes after ejaculation. They can then reach the fallopian tubes, the site of conception, in 30 minutes.

Another caveat for women who want to douche after intercourse is that you must wait if using a spermicidal vaginal contraceptive, because a douche can wash out the spermicide and leave behind live sperm. Vaginal contraceptives usually carry warnings about douching; most recommend waiting at least six hours after intercourse before douching.

Nonoxynol-9 is found in the majority of nonprescription vaginal contraceptives sold in the United States. Examples are Conceptrol (Ortho), a vaginal cream with 5 percent nonoxynol-9; Delfen (Ortho), foam with 12.5 percent; Encare (Thompson Medical),

Properties of vaginal contraceptives

Jelly: *These are water soluble and act as a vaginal lubricant. Some consider them messy.*

Cream: *These are insoluble and should be used primarily with a diaphragm.*

Foam: *These are packaged in pressurized cans and come out like shaving cream. They distribute fairly well in the vagina.*

Suppositories: *These are solid wedges shaped like bullets. They dissolve in the vagina, so must be inserted 10 to 15 minutes before intercourse.*

Contraceptive choices

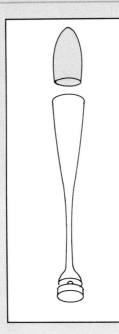

Vaginal suppositories are placed high in the vagina and slowly melt. You should wait 15 minutes after inserting one before having intercourse.

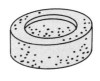

The sponge is pretreated with a sperm-killer, then fitted over the cervix in the vagina. It can be inserted hours before intercourse and must be left in place hours after.

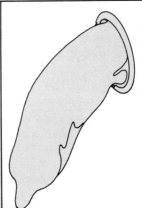

The condom fits over the erect penis. Put it on before intercourse, leaving about ¹/₂ inch at the end to catch the ejaculate.

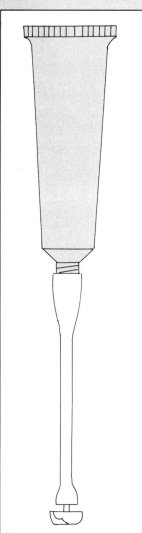

Foam, cream, or jelly is squeezed from a tube into an applicator, which is then placed in the vagina. Pushing down the plunger releases the sperm-killing contraceptive into the vagina around the cervix. The application must be repeated before each act of intercourse.

suppository with 2.27 percent; Emko (Schering), foam with 8 percent; Intercept (Ortho), a suppository with 100 mg of the ingredient; Koromex-A II (Holland-Rantos), jelly with 2 percent; and Ortho-Gynol (Ortho), a jelly with 1 percent.

Octoxynol 9 is more often found in the vaginal jellies and creams that are used with diaphragms, such as Koromex-A II (Holland-Rantos), which has 1 percent of the ingredient.

The newest addition to the vaginal contraceptive category is the sponge. One example is the Today Vaginal Contraceptive Sponge (VLI Corp.). It acts as a physical barrier, much like diaphragm, and is also pretreated with a spermicide.

How to use the rhythm method

To use the rhythm method of birth control, you must determine your fertile period—the period of time when you may become pregnant if you have intercourse. Because every woman's fertile period occurs at a different time, you'll have to figure out your own. You can use an ordinary calendar and pencil:

1. First, determine how long your menstrual cycles last. To do this, mark the day on your calendar that your next menstrual cycle begins—in other words, the day you begin bleeding. Then, do this *every* month for the next 6 months to 1 year. Each cycle begins on the first day of bleeding and ends on the day before bleeding starts again.

2. After you've recorded this for at least 6 months, determine the number of days in your *shortest* cycle. Then subtract 18 from that number. The number you get is the first day of your fertile period. For example, let's say that your shortest cycle lasted 23 days. By subtracting 18 from 23, you get 5. This means that your fertile period begins on the fifth day of your cycle.

3. Next, determine the number of days in your *longest* cycle, and subtract 11 from that number. The number you get is the last day of your fertile period. For example, if your longest cycle is 31 days, subtract 11 from 31. The result is 20. This means that your fertile period ends 20 days after you begin bleeding.

4. Now you know your fertile period, during which you shouldn't have intercourse if you want to avoid pregnancy. Using the figures above as an example, you'd refrain from intercourse from the fifth to the twentieth day of every menstrual cycle for the best chance of avoiding pregnancy.

Understanding your menstrual cycle and your fertile period

Here's what happens during your 28-day menstrual cycle: days 1-13, an egg develops in a follicle in the ovary. On day 14, the follicle bursts, releasing the egg (ovulation). From days 15-28, the egg travels through the fallopian tube to the uterus. If it's fertilized, it attaches to the uterine wall and grows: you're pregnant. If it's not fertilized, the follicle shrivels.

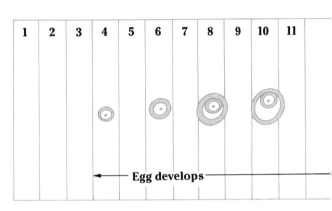

Example of basal body temperature charted through a 28-day cycle

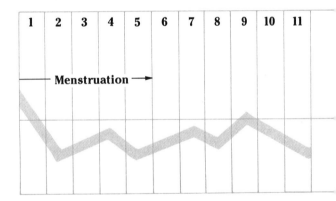

Just before ovulation occurs, your basal body temperature (BBT)—your body temperature when you wake up in the morning—drops slightly. However, when ovulation occurs, your BBT slowly begins to increase. During this time, you should refrain from sexual intercourse. When your BBT stabilizes, you'll be able to safely resume intercourse.

To make this method as successful as possible, you must establish accurate BBTs for each phase of your menstrual cycle. To do this, you must chart your BBT at the same time every morning (about 5 minutes before getting out of bed) for 6 months. For accuracy, use the same thermometer each day. Special thermometers are sold for this purpose.

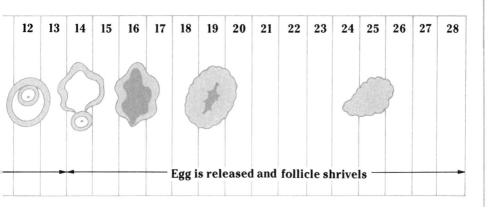

12	13	14	15	16	17	18	19	20	21	22	23	24	25	26	27	28

Egg is released and follicle shrivels

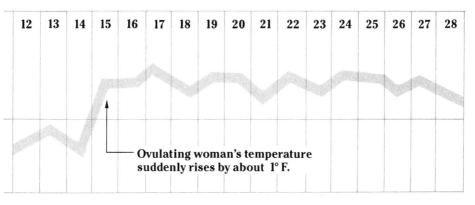

12	13	14	15	16	17	18	19	20	21	22	23	24	25	26	27	28

Ovulating woman's temperature suddenly rises by about 1° F.

You'll need six charts like the example here—one for each menstrual cycle. By connecting the dots indicating each day's BBT, you can easily see when your BBT dropped suddenly, then rose. The rising temperature indicates that ovulation occurred.

After establishing a 6-month pattern, you should note the earliest and latest times ovulation occurred in your cycle. To minimize risk of pregnancy, you must refrain from intercourse for 5 days before the earliest time ovulation occurred and 3 days beyond the latest time. Important: Because this type of birth control isn't reliable until you've established your normal BBT pattern, another form of birth control must be used during the 6-month docu-mentation period.

Several factors may affect your BBT; for example, emotional stress, anxiety, an illness, a disruption in your normal sleeping habits, and using an electric blanket. By raising body temperature, these factors may deceive you into thinking ovulation's already occurred.

8

Cough relievers

Kinds of coughs
Coughs can be productive or nonproductive. A productive cough produces mucus; a nonproductive cough is dry and is therefore sometimes called a hacking cough. You shouldn't use a cough suppressant with a productive cough because coughing up mucus helps clear your lungs.

Coughs both with and without a congested chest are often associated with the common cold. There's nothing worse than feeling a tickle that makes you want to cough. Yet coughing is important—it's a natural, protective reflex that forces fluid or foreign objects out of your lungs, windpipe, and throat. A congested chest can be a sign of a severe cold, asthma, or bronchitis.

There are many reasons why you cough. Some coughs may be a symptom of an oncoming cold or an ongoing allergy or reaction to something in your environment. Others can be a result of smoking or can be linked to emphysema, asthma, pneumonia, heart disease, or lung cancer. It's therefore recommended that you be careful with your cough. If it persists for more than a week, see your doctor. Also see your doctor immediately if you have an accompanying high fever, cough up blood, or have difficulty breathing.

There are more than 800 nonprescription cough relievers available. According to the FDA advisory review panel, cough suppressants should be used only when you want to stifle your impulse to cough, and only when the cough is not accompanied by a congested chest. Cough suppressants are not recommended if you also have a rash or a headache that won't go away. Children under two shouldn't be given cough suppressants.

Oral suppressants
The FDA panel judged three ingredients in cough suppressants as safe and effective: oral codeine, dextromethorphan, and diphenhydramine hydrochloride. Medications for coughs containing these three are called oral suppressants, or antitussives. None will decrease a cough by more than 50 percent, so don't expect it to go away completely. Because it's a narcotic, codeine may not be available in all states as an ingredient in OTC cough remedies. It's generally not addictive when used in small quantities.

Overall, the FDA panel found dextromethorphan, a nonnarcotic, the "drug of choice" when you need an antitussive. In fact, that's the ingredient most nonprescription cough preparations contain. Diphenhy-

How you cough

When you cough, your diaphragm forces out fluid or foreign objects trapped in your airways. Your cough center is in the medulla, which is directly linked to the cerebral cortex in the brain (see star). When any one of your airways—trachea, bronchi, lungs, or nose and throat—is stimulated by too much mucus, your medulla receives a cough message. The medulla then sends this message along to your respiratory muscles and your larynx; then you cough. The respiratory muscles are located behind your rib cage, which is why you can feel them heave when you cough. All this relaying of messages takes place in split seconds.

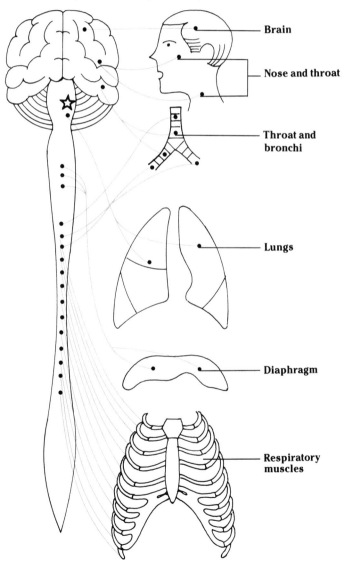

Brain

Nose and throat

Throat and bronchi

Lungs

Diaphragm

Respiratory muscles

dramine hydrochloride, usually available only by prescription, is now found in Parke-Davis' Benylin.

Side effects

Even though these ingredients have been judged safe and effective, they still may produce certain side effects. For example, codeine may cause constipation and nausea and isn't recommended if you suffer from asthma, emphysema, or shortness of breath. Dextromethorphan may cause drowsiness or nausea; diphenhydramine may also cause drowsiness. The latter shouldn't be used if you have glaucoma or problems urinating, nor should you give it to children under six.

The FDA has mandated preparations containing diphenhydramine to carry the following warning: "May cause marked drowsiness. Avoid driving a motor vehicle or operating heavy machinery, or drinking alcoholic beverages."

Alcohol

Many cough syrups contain alcohol, in percentages varying from 1 to 42 percent. For example, Vicks' Formula 44D contains 10 percent alcohol; Chesebrough-Pond's Pertussin 8-Hour Cough Formula, 9.5 percent; and Romilar CF, made by Block, 20 percent. Besides helping to keep all the ingredients mixed, the alcohol may act to depress the central nervous system.

If you're a diabetic or taking sedatives, antidepressants, or any antianxiety medications, you should avoid products with high concentrations of alcohol. Children shouldn't be given these products. Diabetics should be aware of the high sugar content of many OTC cough remedies. Sugar is used because it seems to soothe throats irritated by coughing. If you're a diabetic, choose from many sugar-free medications now available. The FDA panel has identified Ives' Cerose-DM as one such product.

Decongestants

If your cough is producing mucus or phlegm, your body is bringing up fluid from the lungs. It makes no sense to suppress a cough—usually called a "productive" cough—in this case. If the mucus is too thick, drinking plenty of fluids will help thin it out. Most cough medications contain expectorants, which are touted to help thin mucus congestions.

However, the FDA panel rated no expectorant safe or effective for thinning congestion, not even guaifenesin, claimed by some manufacturers to do just that.

Cough syrups and alcohol

When buying a cough syrup for a child be certain to check the ingredients for alcohol. Avoid cough syrups containing alcohol—it can be harmful to children. Keep cough medicines out of children's reach, on the top shelf of the medicine cabinet or with the other poisonous substances in your home.

New studies may yet win it the FDA's safe and effective status. You're probably better off with a combination of one cough suppressant and one oral decongestant to relieve cold symptoms that include a congested chest and cough.

Robitussin-PE (and DM) syrup, manufactured by Robins, and Coricidin cough syrup, made by Schering, are two of many cough medications. Check the label. If the product name is followed by "PE," it contains the decongestant phenylephrine. "DM" stands for dextromethorphan. Decongestants usually help if your cough is caused by a postnasal drip. A cough-cold combination drug product containing an antihistamine isn't recommended for productive coughs because the antihistamine can dry out the mucus.

Increasing the humidity of the air will also help soothe coughs accompanied by congested chests. This can be done by using a steam-mist vaporizer, boiling water, or, in the winter, by placing a pot of water on a steam radiator. In all cases, be careful not to burn yourself with the steam.

Coughs without congestion sound like what you know as "hacking." These are extremely irritable and demand almost immediate soothing. For some, sucking on a piece of hard candy produces enough liquid to bathe the throat and help suppress coughing. Or you can gargle with a mixture of one teaspoon salt in a glassful of warm water. Drinking hot beverages such as

When you need to cough

You take decongestants when you have a chest cold and need to cough productively. Using a vaporizer or standing in a steamy shower may help your decongestant get even better results. Don't take an antihistamine when you have a productive cough because you don't want to dry out your membranes.

Recommended dosages for cough syrups

Adults	Children 6–12:	Children 2–6:	Children less than 2:
One or two teaspoonfuls three or four times a day.	One-half to one teaspoonful three or four times a day.	One-quarter teaspoonful three or four times a day.	Call your doctor.

Always remember to check the label for the manufacturer's guide to dosages.

tea with lemon and honey or hot milk and honey may also help.

Cough drops

Cough drops may provide temporary relief, but none is effective in treating any accompanying cold symptoms. Some cough drops contain an antibacterial agent called cetylpyridinium chloride. Other drops or "medicated lozenges" may contain a surface anesthetic—usually benzocaine—to suppress coughs and soothe the throat. This combination of an anesthetic and cough suppressant in a lozenge is recognized as safe, but the FDA panel found there usually just isn't enough of the suppressant to be effective. Moreover, you should limit your use of an anesthetic because too much may hide symptoms of a more serious illness. Other ingredients include honey, camphor, menthol, and eucalyptus oil—all found safe, but not necessarily effective, by the FDA panel.

FDA approved claims

The FDA has approved these claims as accurate when made for cough suppressants:

"Cough suppressant which temporarily reduces the impulse to cough"

"Temporarily helps you cough less"

"Temporarily quiets cough by its antitussive action"

"The temporary relief of coughs due to minor throat and bronchial irritation as may occur with the common cold or inhaled irritants"

9

Eyes and ears

N o two other organs of the body contribute as significantly to your everyday life as your eyes and ears. The ability to see and hear is something most of us take for granted, but care of our eyes and ears is vital. We're lucky in that our bodies know best how to handle eye and ear problems. For example, your eyes' tears contain an enzyme that combats any bacteria finding their way in.

Eyes

Eye problems are best left to your eye doctor, an ophthalmologist or an optometrist. Even though there are many OTC products for stinging, itchy, red, or blurry eyes, your doctor will know what's best for you. That includes contact lens solutions and cleaners. Some may contain ingredients you might be allergic to.

Eye emergency

If you get a chemical or poison in your eye, you'll have to flush that eye for 15-20 minutes with lukewarm water. Lean over a sink, use a glass, hose, or pail— anything that will hold water—and turn your head so that your untroubled eye is higher than the hurt one. Hold the eyelid away from the eye so the water can flush the poison out from under it. Don't delay! Speed is essential. Washing the eye is more important than calling your doctor. After washing the poison out, go immediately to your eye doctor or the emergency room at your local hospital.

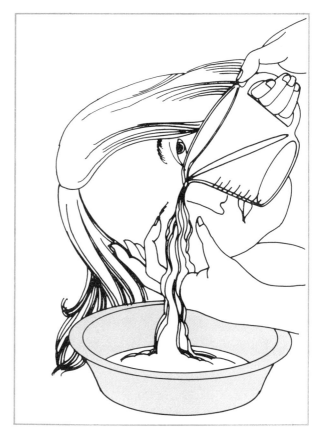

The biggest problem with using nonprescription eye-care products is that you may be tempted to over-use them while the underlying problem causing the symptoms gets worse.

Eyes that itch, burn, and are inflamed may be infected with bacteria or viruses that cause conjunctivitis, or "pinkeye." Sometimes these symptoms are caused by allergies or by swimming in a chlorinated pool. Measles, respiratory infections, rheumatoid arthritis, hyperthyroidism, and diabetes are all diseases that can cause eye trouble. Eyes also react to smog, bright lights, or lack of sleep. Tired eyes can be helped by cold water or cold compresses.

The FDA advisory review panel on OTC Ophthalmic Drug Products was very specific in recommending which eye conditions it considered the consumer able to treat himself with eye drops or ointments. None of these conditions should be self-treated for more than three days. Conditions include:

- tear insufficiency, or "dry eye."

- corneal edema, or swelling. OTC medications are available to treat this condition, but they should only be used with your doctor's permission and supervision.

- foreign bodies in the eye. If a particle cannot be removed with eyewash, see your doctor immediately. Eyewashes should contain only sterile water and a small amount of preservative.

- irritation and inflammation.

The FDA panel approved active ingredients in astringents (to fight bacteria), vasoconstrictors (to shrink swollen vessels), demulcents (to soothe), and emollients (to moisten) in nonprescription drugs you can use for the above eye conditions. Follow directions carefully when you use an eyedropper. Neither a dropper nor a container should ever touch the eye.

Astringents may relieve the hay fever symptoms of eye itchiness and irritation. Zinc sulfate is the only approved active ingredient in eye astringents. Products include BufOpto Zinc Sulfate (Professional Pharmacal).

Four active ingredients in vasoconstrictors may help "get the red out." They are ephedrine hydrochloride (generic); naphazoline hydrochloride, Clear Eyes (Abbott); 0.08 to 0.2 percent phenylephrine hydro-

Glaucoma warning

Glaucoma affects more than 2 million Americans and causes blindness in approximately 15 percent. Doctors don't know why glaucoma occurs. Symptoms include pressure on the eyes, producing blind spots, pain, and redness. You should be tested every year for glaucoma, because it has only occasional symptoms. Unfortunately, these symptoms may be aggravated by nonprescription medications.

Ask your eye doctor if you have acute, or closed-angle, glaucoma, or if you're susceptible to it, because some OTC drugs may cause a first attack or worsen the disease. Be especially wary of antihistamines and vasoconstrictors.

How and when to use an eyewash

You should use an eyewash only when you have a foreign object in the eye, dry eye, or irritation and inflammation. Never overuse this product; if any of these conditions persists, see your eye doctor.

1

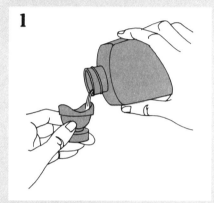

To use an eyewash, fill the cup with the solution.

2

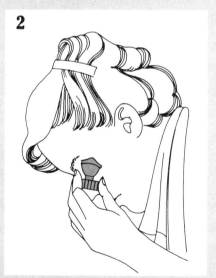

With your head down, place it firmly over your eye.

3

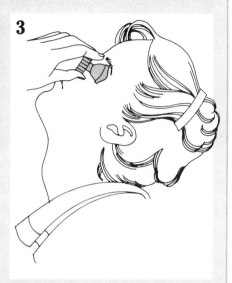

Then tilt your head well back. Open your eye. Look down, to the right, up, to the left.

4

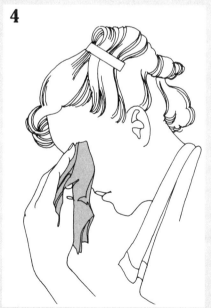

Then lower your head and remove the cup. Blot the excess solution from around your eye.

How to use an eyedropper

To use an eyedropper, first unscrew the top. Squeeze the bulb and put it into the solution. Release the bulb, which will draw the solution up into the dropper. With your head back, hold the dropper over your eye. Look to the left or right, not at the dropper. Then squeeze the bulb slowly to release two or three drops into the eye, being careful not to touch the eye with the dropper.

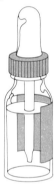

Eye drops in squeeze bottles

Some eye drops come in squeeze bottles; others are in bottles with droppers. Follow directions exactly. Never let the container or the dropper touch your eye.

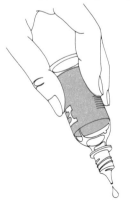

chloride, Isopto Frin (Alcon); and tetrahydrozoline hydrochloride, Visine (Leeming).

Demulcents soothe eyes by keeping in moisture. They're also called artificial tears. The FDA panel found 13 demulcents in eye drops safe and effective:

• carboxymethylcellulose sodium

• hydroxyethylcellulose

• hydroxypropyl methylcellulose

• methylcellulose

• dextran 70

• gelatin

• glycerin

• polyethylene glycol 300

• polyethylene glycol 400

• polysorbate 80

• propylene glycol

• polyvinyl alcohol

• povidone.

Emollients also keep the eyes moist and protect them with an oil-based substance. Lacri-Lube S.O.P ointment (Allergan) is one such product. The FDA panel approved nine emollients in two categories:

1. lanolin preparations, including anhydrous lanolin, lanolin, and nonionic lanolin derivatives.

2. oily ingredients, including light mineral oil, mineral oil, paraffin, white ointment, white petrolatum, and white wax.

Ears

There's some truth to the old adage "Never stick anything in your ear smaller than your elbow." You may be tempted to remove built-up wax with cotton-clad sticks such as Q-Tips (Johnson & Johnson), but you run the risk of pushing the wax farther into the ear canal, thus clogging it.

The FDA panel agreed earwax should be left alone. If you must use anything, make it the end of a finger. Run a washcloth over your outer ear when taking a shower, bath, or washing your face to remove surface dirt.

You may suffer from a tendency to produce and build up a lot of ear wax. Only one active ingredient was judged safe and effective to help you remove accumulated ear wax: 6.5 percent carbamide peroxide in a

Putting in eardrops

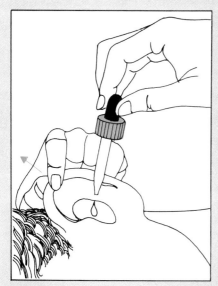

When putting eardrops in your ear, pull the top of the ear up so that the drops go into the ear canal.

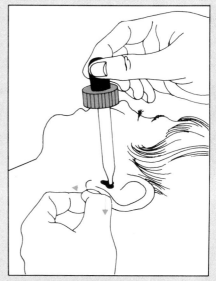

When putting eardrops in a child's ear, pull the ear lobe down and out so that the drops go into the ear canal.

solution of anhydrous glycerin. Debrox (Marion) and Murine Ear Drops (Abbott) both contain this ingredient.

Put the medication into an ear with a dropper and put your head to one side to keep it in. After approximately 15 minutes, gently insert lukewarm water with a small bulb syringe. The water will flush out excess wax and dirt. Don't squeeze the bulb too hard, because a strong water flow could puncture your eardrum.

Earaches, pains, an "underwater" feeling, or leakage from the ears should all be handled by your doctor. These may be symptoms of diseases not directly related to the ears, such as sinus, throat, teeth, gum, or jaw infections. No ear pain relievers were approved by the FDA panel, and, as with eyes, most problems with your ears should be handled by your doctor.

10

Hair and scalp care

FDA-approved claims
The FDA panel found these claims accurate for dandruff products:
"Relieves the itching and scalp-flaking associated with dandruff"
"Relieves the itching, irritation, and skin-flaking associated with seborrheic dermatitis of the scalp and/ or body"
These claims were judged to be false or misleading:
"Guaranteed to control dandruff and scalp itch without shampooing"
"Proteinized formula time-proven to control dandruff"
"An excessive dandruff-control formulation containing a powerful antimicrobial agent"

You may remember this commercial for a leading antidandruff shampoo: a young man is portrayed as highly successful and attractive; others are shown talking to him, but behind his back, they're thinking, "Dandruff." The scourge of popularity and a meaningful social life, dandruff is only too visible in the hair and on one's shoulders.

What causes dandruff? Like everywhere else on the body, when skin dies—as it continually does—the outer layer of dead skin sloughs off. The same process occurs on the scalp. However, here the sebaceous glands produce an oily secretion that is mixed with the dead skin scales, producing dandruff. A normal life cycle for skin cells is 25 to 30 days; dandruff usually occurs when that process is speeded up to 14 days. Dandruff is confined to the scalp, the eyebrows, or both, and only mild redness is apparent.

Dandruff shouldn't be confused with seborrheic dermatitis or psoriasis. Both are considered diseases. In the former case, the scalp is usually very red and itchy, and sometimes the forehead, nose, cheeks, and chest are also involved. This condition requires a doctor's attention.

Psoriasis can be differentiated from dandruff because the scales sit on top of bumps called plaques. It also usually stops at the hairline.

Normal dandruff can be treated with regular shampooing, either several times a week or more if you sweat excessively or work in a big city where there's a

FDA warning

The FDA panel issued the following warning regarding OTC medications used for dandruff and seborrheic dermatitis:

"The panel warns that these products should be kept out of the eyes or rinsed out quickly if they get in, should not be used on children under 2 except as directed by a doctor, and should be kept out of the reach of all children, since some ingredients are poisonous if ingested. If the condition fails to improve or worsens with self-treatment, consult the family doctor or a dermatologist."

lot of environmental pollution. Even if you shampoo every day, it's difficult to harm your hair. You should choose a shampoo product that cleans without removing all the hair's natural oils.

Sometimes, however, excessive flaking occurs. Germs have been ruled out as a cause, so there's no need for shampoos labeled "antiseptic."

The FDA panel has found several ingredients in shampoos effective at controlling dandruff marked by excessive flaking. These include selenium sulfide, available as a 1 percent concentration in Selsun Blue (Abbott). Other ingredients in medicated shampoos include pyrithione zinc, found in Danex (Herbert) and

Understanding dandruff and eczema

Dandruff is a natural flaking off of dead skin cells. The skin combines with scalp oils to form dandruff flakes, as shown in the picture. Dandruff can be worsened by stress, diet, weather changes, and poor hygiene. Shampooing controls dandruff by washing away the dead skin and oil. For some people, more frequent shampooing takes care of dandruff. Others will need a medicated shampoo.

Eczema causes red, itchy, raised patches anywhere on the body. Scratching can damage the skin, thickening and darkening it. Eczema can come and go and is often worse in one season than in others. Its cause unknown, eczema is usually treated with cortisone-type creams.

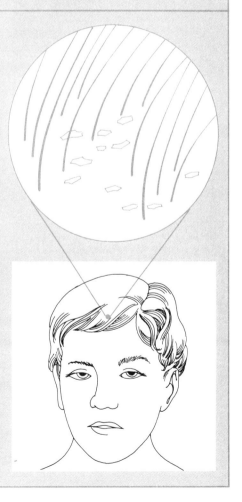

Lice

The head louse is the most common type of louse. It's usually found in the hair and on the scalp. The presence of head lice is usually signaled by head scratching, intense itching, redness, or small bite marks on the scalp. The louse pictured here is greatly enlarged—it's only the size of a pinhead. Lice are parasitic insects

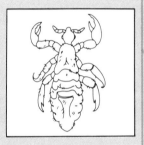

the size of pinheads. They can infest people at all social levels; no one is immune. Lice are easily transmitted from person to person by shared personal articles, such as hats, hair ribbons, combs, towels, and bedding, and by physical contact.

Infestations of lice are easily treated today. Shampoos are sold to be used on infested areas. Along with the shampoo is a fine-toothed comb for removing dead lice and eggs after the treatment. Follow package directions carefully. Don't use these products on eyebrows or eyelashes.

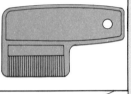

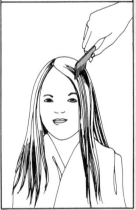

To help prevent reinfestation

If someone in your household or someone you're in close contact with has had lice, certain precautions are necessary to prevent the lice from infesting others. Personal cleanliness and the avoidance of infested persons and their bedding and clothes are most important. These additional steps are also important:

• Change undergarments, clothes, and nightwear daily. Wash in hot water, at least 130° F.

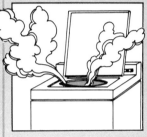

Vacuum upholstered furniture, rugs, and floors frequently. Also, change bedding frequently.

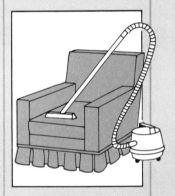

- *Tell children not to use any borrowed combs or brushes and not to wear anyone else's clothes.*

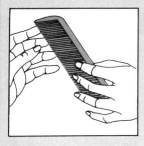

- *Inspect all family members periodically for any new lice infestation.*

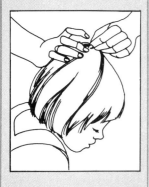

- *Carpets, bedding, furniture, and other objects that become infested can be treated with a spray that will kill the lice but won't harm fabric. The spray is available in drugstores.*

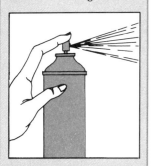

Head & Shoulders (Procter & Gamble); coal tar, found in Tegrin (Block); and sulfur-salicylic combinations, found in Sebulex Medicated (Westwood).

Follow the directions on the product carefully. If you don't, excessive oiliness and a yellowish cast to your hair may result. If one product fails to produce results, try another. It often takes a few tries before your body responds to treatment. These products work better if you suffer from excessive flaking—not just an itchy scalp. The FDA panel could find no scientific basis for an itchy scalp to respond to a medicated shampoo over a regular shampoo.

If, after you've tried a few products, your dandruff gets worse or persists over several weeks, contact your doctor. He or she may be able to prescribe a stronger dose of what's available over-the-counter or may diagnose a condition other than dandruff.

11

Hemorrhoids

Measures for temporary relief from hemorrhoids

• *Ice packs: to alleviate the discomfort of external thrombosed hemorrhoids, apply an ice pack (ice cubes wrapped in a plastic bag will do fine) when the hemorrhoids first appear, and rest in bed. Apply the ice only for a few minutes at a time, and stop applying it altogether after a few hours.*

• *Laxatives can reduce discomfort by softening the stool and keeping the bowels moving. But overuse of laxatives can lead to the very thing they're supposed to correct—constipation. If you rely too much on laxatives, you may never achieve natural regularity. The best policy is to use laxatives only when they're recommended by your doctor.*

• *Enemas may also help reduce discomfort of hemorrhoids, but should only be used at your doctor's recommendation.*

• *Commercial hemorrhoid ointments can soothe raw or burning areas, but they can be expensive and are no more effective than ordinary petroleum jelly.*

• *Witch hazel compresses often will help relieve the pain of hemorrhoids. To make a compress, soak cotton pads in witch hazel.*

Along with dandruff, hemorrhoids enjoy limelight in television, radio, newspaper, and magazine advertisements. You can even find ads in New York City subway cars. It seems ironic that a health problem you can't see yourself without a mirror should be so openly discussed—at least by actors and actresses.

Don't be shy, however, about discussing your anal and rectal problems with your doctor. Sometimes he or she may seem as embarrassed as you feel, for these aren't subjects we grow up discussing easily. The words may be hard to say. Persist. Your health is important, and your doctor can help.

Hemorrhoids involve the anus and the rectum, also known as the anorectal area. The anus is the opening through which your body's solid wastes, or stools, pass. The rectum is the part of the body right above the anus. It's actually part of the lower bowel.

Bleeding, itching, irritation, discomfort, and pain are common symptoms affecting the anorectal area. Hemorrhoids, also called piles, can cause all these symptoms. They're groups of varicose veins that have become swollen and inflamed. It's estimated that one-third of all Americans have them. Most cases begin after age 30.

Hemorrhoids are usually a direct result of chronic constipation. Trying to push out stools can cause the veins to stretch and become packed together. Overuse of laxatives may also be a factor, because of frequent bowel movements. Any change in bowel habits may provoke an attack of hemorrhoids. Just drinking too much alcohol or eating too-spicy food can change bowel habits.

Women frequently get hemorrhoids during or after a pregnancy because of the increased pressure. You're more prone to get them if you have a job where you sit most of the time or are required to stand a lot or lift heavy objects.

Hemorrhoids can occur internally, in the rectum, or externally, around the anus. The internal ones bleed but rarely hurt, because the rectum doesn't have any nerve endings. External ones may not bleed, but can be extremely painful. The pain is because of a vein that has clotted, or stopped up. This is called a thrombosed hemorrhoid. Coughing, sneezing, walking, and sitting can all make the pain worse.

If you notice bright red-colored blood on toilet paper or on your underpants, and you're not menstruating, it's usually the result of the vein rupturing, or splitting, to release the clot. Sometimes this must be done by a physician in order to relieve the pain. All bleeding from the anorectal area, whether new or recurrent, should be reported to your doctor.

The pain of external hemorrhoids may be relieved by taking warm sitz baths (sitting baths). These may also help if you don't have hemorrhoids but suffer from a severe burning and itching sensation caused by in-

Relief from hemorrhoids

Many types of nonprescription drugs can help you treat your anorectal itches and pains. The FDA panel on OTC hemorrhoidal drug products divided these drugs into nine categories based on their ingredients and what symptoms they claimed to relieve.

Name	What it does	Approval
Anesthetics	May help all symptoms.	Three were approved for external use only.
Antiseptics	Clean the area.	None was approved.
Anticholinergics	Block glands activated by nerve endings.	None was approved.
Astringents	Keep bacteria away from the skin.	Two were approved for internal and external use, one for external use only.
Counterirritants	Provide another type of sensation to concentrate on.	One external product was approved.
Keratolytics, or skin-peeling agents	Remove outer layers of dead skin and work best for itching.	Two external products were approved.
Protectants	Provide an outer coating.	Thirteen were approved—12 for internal and external use, one for external use only.
Vasoconstrictors	Help temporarily shrink swollen blood vessels.	Three were approved; two for internal and external use, one for external use only.
Wound-healing agents	Speed the process along.	None was approved.

Sitz baths

Many hemorrhoid sufferers gain relief by sitting in 3 to 4 inches of warm —not hot—water. These baths are especially soothing after bowel movements but may be taken any time. Some people find that adding a few tablespoons of Epsom salts to the bath water brings added relief.

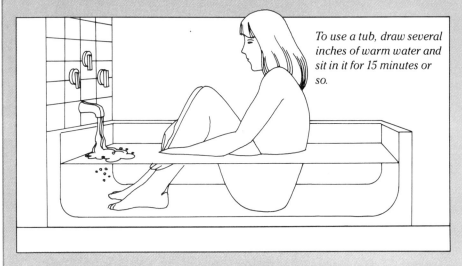

To use a tub, draw several inches of warm water and sit in it for 15 minutes or so.

flamed fissures, or tears, in and around the anus. These also bleed.

To take a sitz bath, fill the bathtub with enough warm water to sit in. Sit in the water for about 15 minutes. Take three or four sitz baths every day.

The baths soothe the inflamed area by relaxing the muscles, called sphincters, around the anus. You can also relieve the pressure by lying down. External hemorrhoids usually clear up by themselves when your bowel movements return to normal. If your hemorrhoids occur internally and then hang out from your anus, they're called protrusions. See your doctor if this happens. You shouldn't try to treat these yourself.

Itching is an anal symptom that can have other causes besides hemorrhoids. The itching may be a skin rash or may be caused by an intestinal infection such as pinworms, common in children. Sometimes it's a side effect of oral antibiotics like ampicillin, lincomycin, or tetracycline. The itching may not appear until a week or two after you stop taking the medication and will disappear by itself, but sometimes it takes a while. Anal itching is also one symptom of diabetes. Even psychological factors can cause itching.

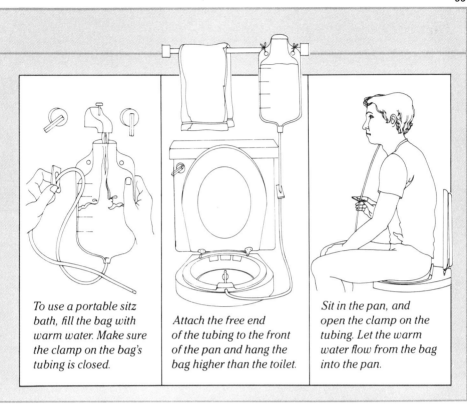

To use a portable sitz bath, fill the bag with warm water. Make sure the clamp on the bag's tubing is closed.

Attach the free end of the tubing to the front of the pan and hang the bag higher than the toilet.

Sit in the pan, and open the clamp on the tubing. Let the warm water flow from the bag into the pan.

Because there can be so many causes of anorectal itching and bleeding, you should be wary of what you try to treat yourself. You're probably safe if the itching, burning, and pain have occurred suddenly, and you don't try to treat them for more than a week. Otherwise, see your doctor. Rectal examinations are recommended annually if you're older than 40, to check for polyps, which are benign tumors, or cancer. Also see the doctor if a child under 12 complains about anorectal problems, because hemorrhoids are rarely the cause. If it's pinworms, children may complain about itching at night.

No nonprescription drug can cure hemorrhoids. At best, different types of products can relieve these symptoms: itching, pain, burning, irritation, discomfort, swelling, and inflammation.

Anorectal OTC products are available in foams, ointments—including creams, gels, and jellies—and suppositories. Some are used externally, around the anus, or anorectally. Others, like suppositories, are pushed through the anus into the rectum, or used intrarectally. The FDA panel found only a few drugs it considered safe and effective when used intrarectally.

Hemorrhoid products

The FDA panel found these active ingredients safe and effective. Each is listed by category and whether the ingredient has been approved for external (anorectal) or internal (intrarectal) use, or both. Check to see whether your symptoms will be relieved by reading the final sentence in each category listing. Brand name products are given randomly as examples; generic means the ingredient is available under that name.

Drug	Trade name and company	External	Internal
Anesthetics Anesthetics relieve burning, itching, discomfort, irritation, and pain. They don't relieve swelling or inflammation.			
benzocaine, polyethylene glycol ointment	Americaine, American Critical Care	●	
hydrocortisone and hydrocortisone acetate	Cortril, Pfipharmecs; Wellcortin, Burroughs Wellcome Co.; Cortaid, Upjohn	●	
pramoxine hydrochloride, cream, 1 percent	Tronothane, Abbott	●	
pramoxine hydrochloride, jelly, 1 percent	Tronothane, Abbott	●	
Astringents Astringents relieve itching, discomfort, irritation, and pain. They may relieve burning. They don't relieve swelling or inflammation.			
calamine (generic)		●	●
witch-hazel water (generic)		●	
zinc oxide (generic)	Zincofax, Burroughs Wellcome Co.	●	●
Counterirritants Counterirritants relieve itching, discomfort, and pain. They may relieve irritation and burning. They don't relieve swelling or inflammation.			
menthol, aqueous solution (generic)		●	

Drug	Trade name and company	External	Internal
Keratolytics Keratolytics relieve only itching.			
alcloxa (generic)		●	
resorcinol (generic)		●	
Protectants Protectants relieve itching, discomfort, irritation, and burning. They may relieve inflammation. They don't relieve pain or swelling.			
aluminum hydroxide gel (generic)		●	●
calamine (generic)		●	●
cocoa butter (generic)		●	●
cod liver oil (generic)	Cod Liver Oil Liquid, Squibb	●	●
glycerin, aqueous solution (generic)		●	
kaolin (generic)		●	●
lanolin (generic)		●	●
mineral oil (generic)		●	●
petrolatum, white (generic)	Vaseline Pure Petroleum Jelly, Chesebrough-Pond	●	●
shark liver oil (generic)		●	●
starch (generic)		●	●
wood alcohols (generic)		●	●
zinc oxide (generic)	Zinc Oxide, Lilly	●	●
Vasoconstrictors Vasoconstrictors relieve itching and swelling. They may relieve pain and discomfort. They don't relieve irritation, burning, or inflammation.			
ephedrine sulfate, aqueous solution (generic)		●	●
epinephrine hydrochloride, aqueous solution (generic)		●	
phenylephrine hydrochloride, aqueous solution (generic)		●	●

12 Mouth care

Sources of bad breath

Bad breath isn't always the result of eating foods like shrimp in garlic sauce. Consider these other common culprits:

- *Cigarettes, cigars, pipes*
- *Alcohol*
- *Sinus infections*
- *Bacteria around teeth*
- *Gum disease*

Bad breath is another scourge of a full social life and getting along at work. For years now, people on television commercials have been prodding one another to be the one to tell the offending party that he or she has "bad breath." Acquaintances have been made and lasting friendships formed on the basis of having fresh-smelling breath—if you believe the ads. In fact, Americans spend approximately $1 million each day to get rid of bad breath.

Bad breath is caused by germs that may be in the back of your throat or on your teeth and gums. It can also be caused by sore throat or sinus infections, or by tooth decay or gum disease. Smoking cigars and cigarettes can leave an unpleasant taste in your mouth and on your breath, as can certain foods like garlic and onions.

Bad breath that doesn't go away is called chronic bad breath, or halitosis. About 10 percent of Americans suffer from halitosis. It's usually a symptom of something else, such as a disease. No amount of mouthwash or candy mints will get rid of it. The remaining 90 percent of Americans who suffer bad breath from time to time can attribute it to bacteria already present in the mouth.

The FDA panel didn't recommend any mouthwashes that contain antimicrobials, or germ-killing agents, because they just don't work. They noted that such products would have to be used repeatedly to control bad breath, and this use might upset the body's natural ability to take care of germs in the mouth. No mouthwash will prevent or cure a cold or sore throat. The best and least expensive mouthwash is a glassful of warm water, gargled. You can add salt or baking soda (sodium bicarbonate).

Mouthwashes won't work on smoker's breath or odors caused by eating garlic and onions because you exhale these odors once they are absorbed by the bloodstream.

Tooth problems

If you have a toothache, it's best to see your dentist. The FDA panel approved only one OTC toothache pain reliever, 85 to 87 percent eugenol in clove or bland oil. However, they noted it should only be used on a tooth the dentist will have to remove anyway, because eugenol attacks a tooth's nerve tissue. These toothaches are extremely painful, with no relief. Until you see a dentist, take an analgesic painkiller and use an ice pack against your face.

No active ingredients were approved in OTC medications marketed as counterirritants, which irritate the gums and get your mind off your aching tooth; or densensitizers, touted to protect highly sensitive—but cavity-free—teeth.

Cavities are caused when bacteria left on teeth produce acid that eats away at enamel covering the teeth. The bacteria form a substance on teeth called plaque.

Fluoride is effective against tooth decay and cavities. Some communities fluoridate the water so all their citizens can benefit. Fluoride is also present naturally in most water. Most toothpastes, gels, and rinses contain fluoride. If a label says "stannous fluoride," it means tin—a common metal—is also included. Tin protects against acid.

Fluoride rinses are different from mouthwashes. They protect the teeth and help prevent cavities. Rinses are swished around in your mouth for about a minute. You should use them once a day. Toothpastes and powders are also called dentifrices. The FDA panel approved acidulated phosphate, sodium, and stannous fluoride as rinses, and sodium monofluorophosphate and sodium and stannous fluoride as dentifrices. Crest with Fluoristat (Procter & Gamble) is a sodium fluoride toothpaste; Colgate is a sodium monofluorophosphate toothpaste.

Your dentist is the best reference for many of your dental care needs, such as how to brush and floss, whether to use waxed or unwaxed floss, a particular brand of toothpaste, tablets that reveal plaque, or even a type of toothbrush. Most dentists recommend brushing after every meal, and daily flossing, too. Be careful not to brush too hard, otherwise your gums might bleed or even recede over time.

Teething relief

The FDA panel found benzocaine to be the only safe and effective ingredient to apply to the gums of teething babies between the ages of four months and two years without consulting a pediatrician. The drug is an anesthetic and decreases pain. It should be applied up to four times a day with a swab. OTC products include Baby Orajel, manufactured by Commerce Drug. Phenol was found safe and effective, but the panel recommended it be used only under the supervision of a doctor.

Cold sores

Other problems involving the mouth for which OTC products are available include cold sores, caused by the herpes simplex type 1 virus. This herpes virus should not be confused with type 2, which causes a genital venereal disease.

Cold sores are also called fever blisters. You usually get them in the corner of the mouth, or above the lips, where they itch and blister. They're very painful and not very attractive. Because they're caused by a virus harbored by your body, they can't be cured or completely prevented. Recurrences usually can be tied to any event that momentarily weakens your body's normal defenses. This can include everything from stress and excitement to sunburn and menstruation. Most cold sores go away by themselves within a week to 10 days, not quick enough for most people. If they don't go away, see your doctor.

One study has found ice effective in preventing recurrences of cold sores. When you feel a cold sore beginning—usually a swelling, burning, and itchy

Benzocaine and cold sores

Analgesics like benzocaine reduce localized pain by numbing nerve endings. Because only the very ending of the nerve is affected, the relief is short-lasting; yet benzocaine produces no ill effects. You can safely reapply it as many times as you like.

What's the difference?

Don't confuse cold sores with canker sores. Canker sores appear inside the mouth as white spots with a red ring around them. The two FDA panels that reviewed OTC products meant for canker sores concluded that none works.

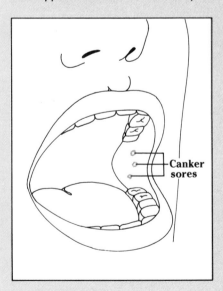

Canker sores

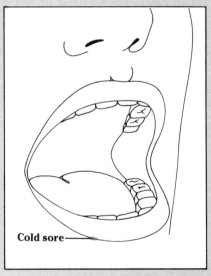

Cold sore

Cold sores and yogurt
Some cold sore sufferers have found sporadic relief from eating yogurt regularly. Some people undergoing antibiotic therapy sometimes develop cold sores during or after the therapy. Since antibiotics kill helpful intestinal bacteria, the yogurt bacteria may be linked to preventing cold sores.

sensation—apply ice against the sore for about five minutes. The area will feel slightly numb. Remove briefly, then reapply. Keep this up for between 45 minutes and two hours. Scientists have found if you do this on the first day you feel the sore, many times it will not erupt and will be gone by the next day.

The FDA panel approved no active ingredients in OTC medications intended to be taken internally for cold sores. However, it did tentatively approve as safe, but not necessarily effective, *Lactobacillus acidophilus* and *Lactobacillus bulgaricus,* bacteria currently sold as products to prevent diarrhea; and lysine monohydrochloride, an amino acid we usually get from food, but which is also available in the form of diet supplements. If you do take the lysine product, don't exceed three grams per day.

Nonprescription products used externally on cold sores are similar to those discussed in the chapters on topicals and hemorrhoids. These products may or may not work against cold sores. They include:

- alcohol
- allantoin
- anhydrous glycerin
- benzocaine
- 0.1 to 3 percent camphor
- lanolin
- 0.1 to 1 percent menthol
- petrolatum
- 0.5 to 1.5 percent phenol
- white petrolatum.

Don't use products containing hydrocortisone or hydrocortisone acetate on cold sores. They may spread the virus rather than curtail it.

Gums

Gums should be considered independently when you're searching for causes of your bad breath. Also called gingiva, the gums are susceptible to gingivitis, a serious disease. This is often caused by plaque, a build-up on your teeth that can escape virtuous brushing and flossing habits and is often a haven for bacteria. Plaque is the primary cause of cavities. Minor irritations to the gums can be caused by too hot food, a slipped toothpick, orthodontic work, or, in babies, new teeth.

The FDA panel categorized five types of OTC medications that may be used to treat gum problems: gingival analgesics, antimicrobial agents, protectants, wound cleansers, and wound-healing agents.

Analgesics are used to reduce pain. One approved active ingredient is benzocaine. It's very effective and is the only analgesic approved for children four months of age or older for teething. It should be applied with a swab. OTC products containing benzocaine include Orajel (Commerce Drug) and Benzodent (Vicks Toiletry Products). Other analgesics include phenol and sodium phenolate, such as Chloraseptic (Procter & Gamble).

Gingival protectants include benzoin tincture (generic) and compound benzoin tincture (generic).

Effective gum wound cleansers are carbamide peroxide in anhydrous glycerin, such as Gly-Oxide Liquid (Marion), or Periolav (Spectru Med); and hydrogen peroxide in an aqueous solution. The latter is available generically or, for example, as PerOxyl Mouthrinse (Hoyt).

The panel found no antimicrobials or wound healers safe and effective for use on gums.

What promotes plaque

Any sort of dietary carbohydrates can contribute to dental plaque. Eating foods between meals — especially those that contain sugar — speeds up the process that promotes plaque. Also, foods that stick to the teeth are more harmful than nonsticky ones. If you do eat sugary, carbohydrate foods such as soft drinks, cakes, and candy bars, try to eat them with a meal and brush afterward. This will lessen their harmful effects because they won't stay on your teeth as long as when you eat them as snacks and don't then brush.

13

Nausea and vomiting

There's nothing worse than feeling you're going to vomit. There's also nothing pleasant about feeling nauseated. *Emesis* is a Greek word meaning "to vomit"; an antiemetic, therefore, is something that prevents nausea and vomiting.

Sometimes, however, vomiting is the body's way of letting us know we've overindulged, eaten some bad food, or may have gotten too much sun. It could also signify pregnancy or a host of diseases, including appendicitis and digestive tract disorders. Prescription drugs such as antibiotics can also upset your stomach.

Motion sickness

For those reasons, the FDA advisory panel recommends that the only nausea you should try to treat yourself is motion sickness. This can include airsickness, carsickness, and seasickness. We feel this way when our sense of balance is disturbed. Often it's accompanied by dizziness.

According to the FDA review, only three active ingredients found in antiemetics are safe and effective in aiding against motion sickness. They are dimenhydrinate, cyclizine, and meclizine. All are antihistamines. Side effects of these drugs include a dry mouth, blurred vision, and often some drowsiness. None should be taken with alcohol or prescription drugs such as sedatives, otherwise drowsiness may be pronounced. Driving a car or operating heavy equipment or machinery is also not recommended. Young children should take only products containing dimenhydrinate, such as Dramamine.

Pregnant women can use antiemetics, but these products are neither approved nor considered safe for the nausea and vomiting associated with early pregnancy's "morning sickness." Antiemetics containing two of the recommended effective ingredients, meclizine and cyclizine, have been found to cause fetal abnormalities in experimental animals. They may therefore be hazardous to the fetus, especially in the first few months of pregnancy.

Brand names of drugs containing 25 mg of meclizine include Antivert and Bonine. Marezine HCl tablets contain 50 mg of cyclizine.

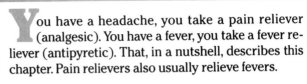

14 Pain and fever relievers

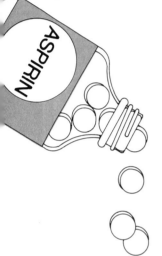

Aspirin and ibuprofen
People who are allergic to aspirin will probably have a reaction to ibuprofen.

You have a headache, you take a pain reliever (analgesic). You have a fever, you take a fever reliever (antipyretic). That, in a nutshell, describes this chapter. Pain relievers also usually relieve fevers.

Aspirin

Aspirin, which has been around the longest of all analgesics, is also the most common of all nonprescription drugs. It comes in many forms, from plain or buffered tablets to liquids and effervescent tablets. It's available alone, or in combination with other analgesics, antacids, or even decongestants.

Aspirin reduces aches, pain, and fever in many common illnesses. It can help you battle a cold or the flu, or muscle or joint pains. In some cases, it also works for women who have mild menstrual cramps. Those suffering from chronic rheumatoid arthritis and osteoarthritis can also use it because it has an anti-inflammatory effect.

But aspirin and all its competitors won't work for all symptoms and in some cases can't be tolerated by all people. For example, migraine sufferers and others who experience severe pain are usually not helped by any form of aspirin. Some people are allergic to aspirin, which may aggravate asthma or cause hives or a skin rash. Liver damage is possible, as is kidney damage, if too much is taken with laxatives.

Sometimes extended use of aspirin may result in anemia, because small amounts of blood are lost daily through irritation of the stomach lining. Greater irritation can cause peptic or bleeding ulcers. The FDA panel warns not to take any analgesic for more than ten days. Overdosage of aspirin may also cause ringing in the ears. Hearing loss may follow, which is reversible if the dosage is reduced.

The blood's ability to clot may be slowed by aspirin, which is why patients facing surgery should stop taking aspirin at least one week before their operation. Be sure to tell your doctor of your medication.

For all these reasons, aspirin is not recommended if you're taking anticoagulants, antidiabetic medication, or arthritis drugs. What makes aspirin work may interfere with the actions of other drugs. Children with flu or chicken pox should not be given aspirin because it may be associated with Reye's syndrome, a rare and fatal childhood disease. It has been found to affect children between the ages of six months and 15 years who are recovering from the chicken pox or flu.

Another form aspirin takes is as an ingredient in effervescent tablets such as Alka-Seltzer. Two tablets dissolved in a glass of water provide relief from mild-to-moderate pain. It should not be used in this form too frequently, however, because it disrupts digestion. In addition, its high bicarbonate content may cause gastric irritation. Its high salt content should be avoided by anyone on a sodium-restricted diet.

Other ingredients

The FDA has banned some ingredients that used to be combined with aspirin because of their side effects. One you should be wary of is phenacetin. A product called A.P.C. used to be widely sold; its three active ingredients were aspirin, phenacetin, and caffeine. In 1973, however, Canada banned the sale of drugs combining phenacetin with aspirin because the combination had been linked to kidney damage. Although phenacetin has been banned, some products containing the substance may still be on store shelves or in your medicine cabinet. Avoid buying it, and throw away any product you still might have with phenacetin in it.

Another ingredient in OTC analgesics the FDA recalled is methapyrilene. The National Cancer Institute reported in 1979 that the substance caused liver cancer in rats and mice. The FDA agreed. If you have any old medication around, check it for methapyrilene.

The FDA advisory panel on internal analgesics notes that the fewer ingredients in OTC drugs the better. They recommend that "no more than two safe and effective analgesics" be used in one product. These combination products may expose you to potential side effects of both or all ingredients. Studies have yet to show that the sum of many different analgesic parts is greater than the whole for treating symptoms.

Caution

Don't mix ibuprofen with either aspirin or acetaminophen without your doctor's advice.

Ibuprofen

One new entry into the analgesic market is ibuprofen, sold as Advil or Nuprin. Ibuprofen is a drug that has been reclassified by the FDA from a prescription to a nonprescription status. It's indicated "for the temporary relief of minor aches and pains associated with the common cold, headache, toothache, muscular aches, backache, for the minor pain of arthritis, for the pain of menstrual cramps, and for reduction of fever." It's available in coated tablets.

Although products containing ibuprofen don't contain aspirin, warnings about similar side effects appear on the label. Follow these recommendations. Taking the product with milk may prevent heartburn or other stomach problems.

If you can't take aspirin or ibuprofen, then acetaminophen is recommended. Besides Tylenol, brand names include Datril, Liquiprin, and Tempra. Acetaminophen has the same ability as aspirin to relieve minor pains and fevers. However, because it has no anti-inflammatory properties, it really won't relieve muscle aches or menstrual cramps. Like most drugs, even acetaminophen is potentially dangerous. Large doses may cause death from liver damage.

15

Skin products

Where acne appears
Acne often appears along the hairline, on the cheeks, and sometimes on the chin. Acne doesn't always confine itself to the face; it can appear on the upper back and shoulders, upper arms, and chest.

Diet and acne
The connection between diet and acne has become a controversial issue. Dermatologists aren't as strict about diet as they were in former years, but many still recommend cutting down, as far as possible, on fatty foods such as milk, butter, ice cream, french-fried potatoes, salad dressing, mayonnaise, potato chips, peanut butter, pizza, and chocolate. Diet has become less stressed in acne treatment because now we know that the disorder results from a variety of factors.

In general, fresh foods, properly prepared—raw, if appropriate—moderate in amount, low in fat and sugar content, and high in vitamin and mineral content, promote healthy skin and a healthy body.

Topicals are applied to the skin to treat or protect it. Many common skin conditions such as acne, athlete's foot, calluses, corns, warts, burns, and sunburns can be treated with topical medications. Topicals can also prevent harm, as is the case with sunscreens.

Acne

Acne is the bane of existence of many—if not all—adolescents. As time goes by, more and more myths are dispelled about what does and doesn't cause acne. For example, chocolate, junk foods, amount of sexual activity, and cleanliness are no longer believed to have anything to do with acne.

When sex hormone production increases in adolescence, it stimulates acne. What's involved are the sebaceous glands, which produce an oily substance called sebum. Sebum flows outward to the skin, where it may get plugged up in a pore. In its earliest stage, it's a whitehead. When more dead skin cells accumulate and are pushed outward, it becomes a blackhead. Finally, if germs enter the picture, pus is formed from white blood cells that died trying to fight the germs.

You shouldn't attempt to treat acne yourself if you're over 30, pregnant, or your acne appears to be producing large cysts that leave scars. In these cases, consult a dermatologist.

The only approved OTC active ingredient for treating acne is benzoyl peroxide. It has been used in many medications since the 1920s. Because it may cause some irritation, however, the FDA panel requires products containing this ingredient to carry the following warning: "Persons with very sensitive skin or a known allergy to benzoyl peroxide should not use this medication. If uncomfortable irritation or excessive dryness and/or peeling occurs, reduce the frequency of use or the amount of dosage. If excessive itching, redness, burning, or swelling occurs, discontinue use. If these symptoms persist, consult a doctor promptly. Keep away from the eyes, lips, and other mucous membranes. Some preparations may bleach hair or dyed fabrics."

Examples of OTC products containing benzoyl peroxide are Oxy 10 (Norcliff Thayer), Benoxyl 10 (Stiefel),

How a pimple forms

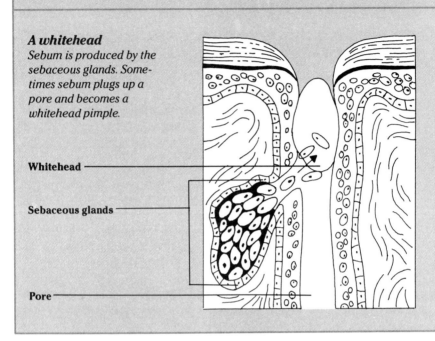

A whitehead
Sebum is produced by the sebaceous glands. Sometimes sebum plugs up a pore and becomes a whitehead pimple.

Whitehead

Sebaceous glands

Pore

Comedone extractor
Squeezing pimples is never a good idea. Bacteria and infection may spread, causing new pimples to form and possibly causing scars. Never use a comedone extractor. If you have a pimple that is painful or that you think needs to be drained, see your dermatologist.

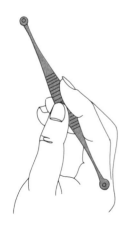

and Clearasil BP Acne Treatment (Vicks Toiletry Products). These products are available as lotions, creams, gels, sticks, ointments, soaps, or medicated pads.

As with many other drug combinations, the fewer active ingredients in one product, the better. For that reason, the FDA panel approved only one combination product and an equivalent variant of that: a combination of sulfur 8 percent and resorcinol 2 percent; and the combination of sulfur 8 percent plus resorcinol monoacetate 3 percent. Interestingly, neither ingredient was approved by the FDA panel on its own because of doubts about both safety and effectiveness. Medications containing this combination include Acnomel (Menley & James).

Some active ingredients were conditionally approved. These include povidone-iodine and salicylic acid.

The FDA panel advised cautious use of what's known as a comedones extractor, a pimple-squeezing device that can be bought at a drugstore.

Athlete's foot
Athlete's foot, jock itch, and ringworm are all caused by fungi, or molds. They like to grow in warm, moist areas on the body—between the toes, under the arms,

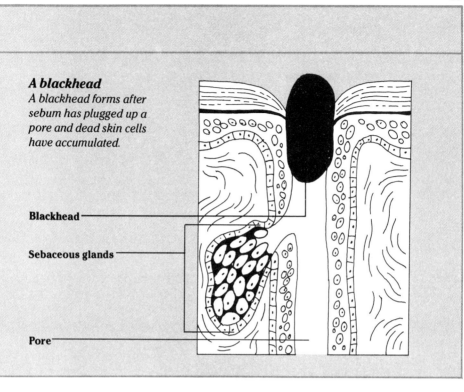

A blackhead

A blackhead forms after sebum has plugged up a pore and dead skin cells have accumulated.

Blackhead

Sebaceous glands

Pore

and in the crotch area. Their presence is usually marked by redness and itching. There may be some pain and cracking of the skin, and there may be a rotting smell.

All these fungi, no matter on what part of the body they exist, respond essentially to the same treatment. The FDA panel noted that unlike most OTC drugs, antifungals actually treat the disease, not just the symptoms. They recommend that before treatment, the affected area be washed and dried. Then you should apply the antifungal twice, in the morning and at night.

The panel cautioned that fungus infections shouldn't be taken lightly. Without proper treatment, they may cause a greater illness in the body; the drugs may also be absorbed by the body in too great quantities. For that reason, it's recommended that you give yourself two weeks to clear up jock itch and a month for athlete's foot and ringworm. After that, see a doctor, or, at the very least, switch products.

Antifungals are available as creams, powders, liquids, ointments, and aerosol sprays. The panel found it's more difficult for the drug to reach the fungus when it's in the form of a cream, powder, or ointment, so a liquid is better.

Athlete's foot

Athlete's foot is a fungal infection. It may be contracted in public shower rooms or result from your feet being cooped up in moist places for too long.

Approved active ingredients for treatment of jock itch, athlete's foot, and ringworm include haloprogin, iodochlorhydroxyquin, miconazole nitrate, tolnaftate, and undecylenic acid and its salts; calcium undecylenate, copper undecylenate, and zinc undecylenate. Cruex (Pharmacraft) contains undecylenic acid and its salts; Tinactin (Schering) has tolnaftate.

Calluses, corns, and warts

It makes sense that a product conditionally approved by the FDA panel for use on acne of the face is also approved as safe and effective in removing calluses and corns: salicylic acid. It causes the skin to peel.

Calluses usually appear on the bottom of the feet and are hard. Corns are more likely to be found on the toes and may be hard or soft or a combination of the two. Both are caused primarily by friction or pressure, such as from shoes that are too tight or socks that rub. When you try to get rid of corns and calluses, it also makes sense to eliminate these frictions. Otherwise, the problem will recur.

Salicylic acid is available in many different forms: a collodion, which is a solution that is applied wet and leaves behind the active ingredient when it dries; a foot salve, or ointment; and medicated disks, pads, and plasters, all of which contain the medication on a form of bandage placed over the corn or callus.

Examples of products approved by the FDA panel include Mediplast (Beiersdorf), and "2" Drop Corn/Callus Remover (Scholl's).

Warts are also treated well with salicylic acid, provided you treat only common and plantar warts yourself. These can appear on the hands, face, feet, and sometimes other parts of the body. They aren't dangerous, merely ugly and embarrassing. Unlike calluses and corns, which are caused by external pressures, warts are caused by viruses.

Common warts are usually gray in color, small, and resemble cauliflower. Plantar warts are found only on the soles of the feet and are flat. If you have a wart you don't think fits into either category, consult a doctor. You may have a wart that needs to be cut out surgically, or it may not be a wart but skin cancer.

Treatment for warts is called wart paint. The active ingredient used to kill the warts must be kept from the surrounding normal tissue. By "painting" the medication on the wart, you can control exactly where it goes.

Corns

Corns are usually found on the toes and can be hard or soft. They're caused primarily by friction or pressure; for example, from wearing too-tight shoes.

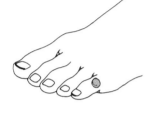

Corn removers

The FDA panel made this warning about callus and corn removers:

"Do not exceed five treatments. Do not use if you are a diabetic or have poor blood circulation, because serious complications may result. Do not use on irritated skin or if the area is infected or reddened."

Common wart

Common warts can develop singly or in groups and may appear on any part of the body—they usually occur on the hands. Common warts are raised, have rough surfaces, are gray in color, and vary in size from as tiny as a matchhead to approximately an inch in diameter.

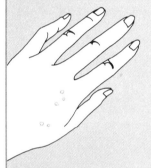

Inside a common wart

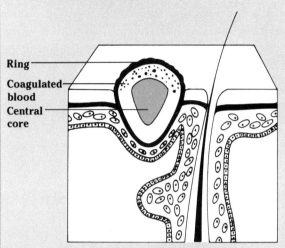

Ring
Coagulated blood
Central core

Inside a common wart is a soft, central core surrounded by a firm ring resembling a callus. Multiple tiny black dots on the surface are bits of coagulated blood in the wart.

Wart removers

The FDA panel had this to say about wart removers:

"Wart-remover drug products should not be used on moles, birthmarks, or unusual warts with hair growing from them, because precancerous and cancerous growths may be mistaken for warts. Use of these products will aggravate these conditions. If treatment has not succeeded after 12 weeks, discontinue the over-the-counter medication and see a doctor."

Plantar warts

Plantar warts are caused by the common wart virus. Since they usually appear on the points of pressure on the sole of your foot, they'll make walking painful or impossible, and you'll need immediate treatment for them.

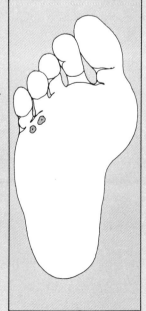

Besides salicylic acid, the FDA panel found three combinations as conditionally approved:

- salicylic acid (5 to 17 percent) and lactic acid (5 to 17 percent) in a collodion base
- salicylic acid (5 to 17 percent) and glacial acetic acid (11 percent) in a collodion base
- ascorbic acid (0.16 percent) and calcium pantothenate (0.20 percent)

Products containing salicylic acid include Wart-Off (Pfipharmecs) and Off-Ezy (Commerce Drug).

Skin protectants

Skin protectants are different from most OTC medications because instead of being used to relieve a symptom, they're used to create a barrier between the skin and the world's irritants. These irritants include wetness, dryness, chemicals, or the pressure and rubbing of clothes or bandages. These topicals can be lubricants, enhance moisture retention, or even soften the skin. Their uses include protection from burns and wound healing.

The rays of the sun
Remember that the sun's rays are strong enough to tan or burn you even on cloudy, foggy, or hazy days. Sand, water, and cement reflect the sun's rays. Even in the water or under a beach umbrella you're protected from only about 50 percent of the dangerous rays.

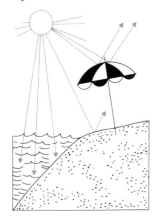

Burn depths

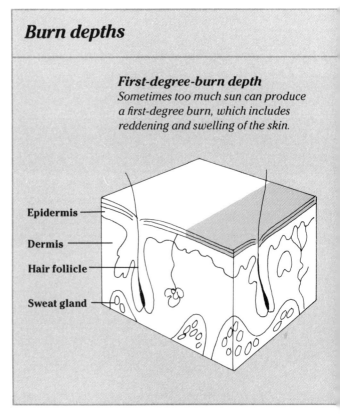

First-degree-burn depth
Sometimes too much sun can produce a first-degree burn, which includes reddening and swelling of the skin.

Epidermis

Dermis

Hair follicle

Sweat gland

Burns

You should treat only first- and second-degree burns—including sunburns—by yourself. In first-degree burns, the skin is red; in second-degree burns, the outer layer of the skin is destroyed and may be blistered. Initial treatment for all burns is to place the surface in cold water. Avoid using running water, which can add to pain, or ice cubes, which are too cold. If you don't have a place to soak the burned surface, substitute cold compresses from which the water has been wrung out. Continue for 20 to 30 minutes. Cover with a skin protectant.

FDA panel-approved skin protectants include allantoin, aluminum hydroxide gel, calamine (prepared calamine and calamine lotion), cocoa butter, cornstarch, dimethicone (dimethyl polysiloxane), glycerin (glycerine and glycerol), kaolin, petrolatum preparations (petrolatum and white petrolatum), shark-liver oil, sodium bicarbonate, zinc acetate, zinc carbonate, and zinc oxide. Almost all of these products are available in a generic form.

Caution

Don't apply butter, lard, or oil to a burn. Instead, use cold water.

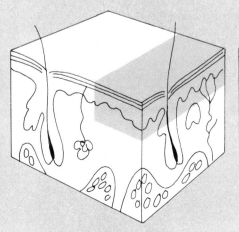

Second-degree-burn depth
Second-degree burns are more serious, producing blisters that may be either superficial or deep. Such burns can usually heal themselves.

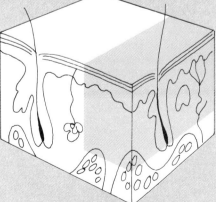

Third-degree-burn depth
Third-degree burns are potentially life-threatening. They destroy skin, fat, even bone; scarring is unavoidable.

No active ingredients were approved as safe and effective wound healers. This includes aloe vera, a product used by some to relieve sunburn pain.

Diaper rash and prickly heat

Diaper rash is one malady that benefits from the use of skin protectants. It's caused by feces and urine, which irritate the skin. Another rash caused by excess heat and trapped moisture is called prickly heat, or miliaria. It's marked by red bumps that may itch or sting your baby. These bumps are sweat glands that erupt on adjacent skin when clogged with water, feces, or urine. Other contributors to diaper rash and prickly heat are soaps and detergents used to clean cloth diapers.

To treat simple diaper rash, frequent washing and diaper changing is recommended. Also, if your baby is in a cloth diaper, switch to a plastic-backed disposable one, or vice versa. Sometimes a change is all that's needed. When possible, leave the diaper off so the irritated skin can get some air.

The FDA panel recommended that after you've washed your baby use skin protectants such as petroleum jelly and cornstarch, already routinely used by many people, before you apply a diaper.

If diaper rash or prickly heat doesn't clear up in a couple of days, consult your pediatrician. The rash may be the symptom of a medical problem such as a milk allergy.

Sunscreens

One topical that no one should do without is a good sunscreen. Although suntans are often associated with good health and vigor, long-term effects of too much sun—besides an initial sunburn—can include premature aging and wrinkling of the skin and cancer. According to the American Cancer Society, about one in every seven Americans has skin cancer, and people are developing it at a younger age.

Fortunately, you can prevent much of the sun's damage by applying sunscreens. Sunscreens block out ultraviolet—or UV—rays in sunlight. You can't see these rays. Most sunscreens protect only against ultraviolet B (UVB) rays. These are the rays primarily responsible for sunburn. However, studies are now showing that ultraviolet A (UVA) rays may be what contribute to aging the skin. To protect yourself, use a new "broad spectrum" sunscreen, such as Shade (Plough) or Block Out (Sea & Ski). You probably won't tan as quickly as you

Protection for infants
The FDA panel has approved these skin protectants for use on infants' skin without medical supervision.

- *allantoin*
- *aluminum hydroxide gel*
- *calamine*
- *cocoa butter*
- *cornstarch*
- *dimethicone*
- *glycerin*
- *petrolatum preparations (petrolatum, white petrolatum)*
- *sodium bicarbonate*
- *zinc carbonate*
- *zinc oxide*

All may be used on infants from birth except aluminum hydroxide gel and glycerin. You should wait until a child is six months old before using these products.

Phenol should never be used for diaper rash.

A common skin problem for babies
Diaper rash produces reddening and soreness of a baby's skin in the areas usually covered by a diaper. This skin irritation develops on a baby's buttocks, in the anal area, around the genitals, on the upper thighs, and on the lower abdomen. Usually caused by wet diapers, it tends to recur.

normally would when you also protect against UVA rays.

The FDA panel approved some 20 active ingredients in sunscreens. The most common, however, is para-aminobenzoic acid—or PABA—and its derivatives. Used correctly, sunscreens allow you to stay in the sun longer without burning. This is one case where you can't apply too much. For best results, apply a sunscreen from 30 minutes to two hours before you plan to sunbathe.

Photosensitivity

Some prescription drugs may cause what's called a photosensitivity reaction in your skin when you go out in the sun. The skin may redden worse than a sunburn, blister, and peel, or you may get an allergic reaction, like a rash. Sunscreens aren't always reliable in preventing a photosensitive reaction, although they do provide some protection. Be especially cautious if you're taking oral antibiotics such as demeclocycline, doxycycline, or tetracycline. Large doses of vitamin A, sometimes prescribed for acne, are also a photosensitizer, as is the tranquilizer chlorpromazine. Check with your doctor if you're taking a prescription drug and you're not sure about its effects.

Sun protection factor

The numbers you see on sunscreen products—usually from 2 to 15—are a direct result of the FDA panel's recommendations. It developed a system called Sun Protection Factor (SPF) to measure the effectiveness of sunscreen products. Generally, the number tells you by how much the product increases your skin's natural sun protection. The SPF you choose will depend on your skin type.

Skin type	Recommended SPF
Burns easily; never tans	8 or higher
Burns easily; tans minimally	6 to 7
Burns moderately; tans gradually	4 to 5
Rarely burns; always tans well	2 to 3
Rarely burns; tans easily	2

16 Sleep aids and stimulants

If you eat the right foods, drink plenty of water, exercise, and get enough sleep every night, chances are you'll never need to use a sleep aid, or sedative, or a stimulant. Sedatives relax your body and can help you sleep; stimulants pep you up. The most common stimulant—and the only approved active ingredient—is caffeine.

The FDA panel found no active ingredients safe and effective when used as a daytime sedative. In fact, the FDA ordered removed from the marketplace all sedatives sold for daytime use. If you're anxious, nervous, tense, feel stress, and are having trouble getting through the day, see your doctor. You're better off in this case with a prescription product taken under your doctor's supervision.

If you have occasional trouble falling or staying asleep, however, there's no harm in careful use of non-prescription sleep aids. All such products should be used only by adults, and not for longer than two weeks at a time.

Most sleep aids contain antihistamine, also found in cold preparations. Antihistamines reverse the action of histamines, naturally produced substances. A by-product or side effect of this action is drowsiness. Sleep aids shouldn't be taken with alcohol. You should also not take them if you have glaucoma, an enlarged prostate, asthma, heart disease, or a peptic ulcer; nor should you give them to children under 12.

If you take antihistamine-based OTC medications to help you sleep, you should be aware of certain side effects, including tiredness, blurry vision, dizziness, or even nausea, vomiting, constipation, and diarrhea. Don't drive after taking these drugs.

The antihistamines diphenhydramine; diphenhydramine hydrochloride (Sominex tablets, Beecham Products); diphenhydramine monocitrate; and doxylamine succinate are the only active ingredients approved by the FDA panel for use in sleeping aids. Pregnant and breast-feeding women should not use doxylamine succinate (Unisom, Leeming).

Many products contain pyrilamine maleate. This antihistamine has been found safe and effective when used for colds but not when it's used to help you sleep.

That's because it can cause side effects, such as nausea and vomiting, that would certainly interfere with your sleep. Most companies use the drug as a substitute in products they previously manufactured with the drug methapyrilene. This drug was banned after it was found to cause cancer in laboratory animals.

Stimulants

Stimulants are drugs to help keep you awake when you're feeling tired but don't want to sleep. Sometimes you may want to stay up to finish some extra work or a term paper, or if you have a long drive home.

The FDA panel decided stimulants cause no harm if you use them only occasionally. Manufacturers of stimulants can accurately claim their products "help restore mental alertness or wakefulness when experiencing fatigue or drowsiness." As noted, the only approved ingredient is caffeine. Recommended doses are 100 mg to 200 mg every three to four hours. This equals about one cup of coffee, so don't combine the OTC drugs with this brew or with tea or soft drinks. Too much caffeine can make you nervous and edgy and can give you headaches.

Caffeine tablets and capsules can be bought generically, or as No Doz (Bristol-Myers) or Quick Pep (Thompson). Don't take caffeine in these forms for more than a couple of weeks, and don't give them to your children. Stimulants shouldn't be taken to combat the effects of alcohol or for a hangover. The combination could make you sick.

17

Sore throats

More people go to a doctor for a complaint of "sore throat" than for any other symptom. A mild sore throat can be caused by yelling, too much talking, or smoking. Usually, however, a sore throat is a symptom tied to an infection or other disease, sometimes one as serious as cancer. For those reasons, the FDA panel on OTC Oral Cavity Drug Products warns: "Severe or persistent sore throat accompanied by high fever, headaches, nausea, and vomiting may be serious. Consult a physician promptly. Do not use these drugs for more than two days or administer to children under 3 years of age unless directed by a physician."

"These drugs" refers to those whose ingredients were found safe and effective by the FDA panel. You can buy them as mouthwashes, gargles, sprays, lozenges, powders, drops, and chewing gum. The panel found sprays to be slightly more effective than gargles. As with bad breath, a good remedy for a sore throat is to gargle with warm water.

What's approved

The panel divided sore mouth and throat medicines into seven categories. Their approved active ingredients follow.

1	Anesthetics/ analgesics	aspirin (in gum), benzocaine, benzyl alcohol, dyclonine hydrochloride, hexylresorcinol, menthol, phenol, salicyl alcohol, sodium phenolate.
2	Antimicrobials	no active ingredients were judged both safe and effective.
3	Astringents	alum, zinc chloride.
4	Debris removers	carbamide peroxide, sodium bicarbonate.
5	Decongestants	no active ingredients were judged both safe and effective.
6	Demulcents	elm bark, gelatin, glycerin, pectin.
7	Expectorants	no active ingredients were judged both safe and effective.

18

Weight-control products

Make your own
Most appetite suppres-
sants help you control the
amount you eat by making
you feel full. (You take the
suppressant at a set time
before you eat.) You can
make your own suppressant
by adding a couple of table-
spoons of bran to a glass of
vegetable juice. Drink this
30 minutes before a meal: it
will decrease your hunger.

A body considered "sexy" in the 1950s would be too fleshy by today's thin standards. We're constantly bombarded in advertising and on television by society's notion of the perfect figure, often reed thin. In the search for perfection, however, you should never lose sight of the importance of your good health.

The best way to lose weight is to reduce your intake of calories and to increase your level of activity. There are really no shortcuts. Any diet that allows you to lose more than one or two pounds a week is probably not healthy. If you want to lose more, start a diet on your own, or gain weight, always consult a doctor first. Even the Weight Watchers® program requires a doctor's signature of consent before you can begin. If you have high blood pressure or kidney or heart disease, you shouldn't attempt to lose weight on your own.

There's good reason for this. Many people can become obsessed with wanting to fit in with the stereotyped notion of what's beautiful. As a result, many women—and men—are literally starving themselves into shape, or binging on food and then purging it. Medical terms for these two eating disorders are anorexia nervosa and bulimia. In both cases, the reward may not only be desired thinness but an inability to quit there. Heart trouble and death can result from placing too much stress on your body without providing essential nutrients.

Appetite suppressants

If you have only a few pounds to lose and you get your doctor's go-ahead, there are many nonprescription drugs that can help you achieve your goal. Most of these control your hunger. You take them before your regular meals, so you feel full, eat less, and thus lose weight. These are called appetite suppressants. They're available in the form of capsules, powders, liquids, drops, and chewable squares resembling pieces of candy.

Sometimes diet aids are complete meals in the form of liquids, soups, powders, or cookies. They're usually nutritionally balanced, calorie-controlled substitutes for solid food and should only be used temporarily. If you want to use them longer, get your doctor's consent

Avoiding misleading claims

The FDA panel agreed what weight-reducing products can and can't claim to do. It found the following claims to be accurate.

"Appetite control to aid weight reduction"

"Helps curb appetite"

"Use as an adjunct to diet control"

"Appetite depressant in the treatment of obesity"

"An aid in the control of appetite"

These claims by manufacturers, however, could not be proved.

"Provides bulk to add to low caloric intake and helps to satisfy the feeling of hunger caused by emptiness"

"Contains one of the most powerful diet aids available without prescription"

"The delightful aid to appetite control"

"Easy-to-follow reducing plan built around food you love to eat. You will eat well but less and lose weight without going hungry"

"Get rid of unsightly bulges"

"The modern aid to appetite control"

"Now enjoy a slim, trim figure. Lose pounds. Reduce inches"

"Lose weight starting today.... Look your best, feel your best"

"Delightfully delicious, scientifically formulated to help you control your appetite quickly, pleasantly"

"Trims pounds and inches without crash diets or strenuous exercise"

and ask him or her to supervise your weight loss. One side effect of these products is bowel irregularities.

Artificial sugars

Other weight-control aids that you may not even think about are the artificial sugars: saccharin and aspartame. Cyclamate, banned by the FDA in 1970 after studies implicated it as causing cancer in laboratory animals, may make a comeback. None of these artificial sweeteners is completely without risk. Your best bet is to limit consumption of these sweeteners and products containing them.

Aspartame, sold under the name NutraSweet

Banned products

Artificial sweeteners haven't had it easy. In 1970, the FDA banned cyclamate because it was found to cause cancer in laboratory animals. However, it may make a comeback. The FDA's cancer assessment committee recently gave cyclamate a favorable report, and the National Academy of Sciences is now reviewing the data. Cyclamate's return remains controversial.

In 1977, the FDA imposed a ban on saccharin. However, the ban was placed under a moratorium by Congress that has since been renewed three times and will probably go for a fourth. Although initial studies showed saccharin caused cancer in laboratory rats, there's some dispute about imposing a complete ban based on these results alone.

(Searle), is the newest artificial sweetener. Many consider its taste closest to sugar, although it's about 180 times sweeter. Initial studies of this product are also controversial: some claim it causes brain tumors in rats, and depression, sleeping problems, headaches, and seizures in humans; other studies find no such links. Both sides agree, however, that if you have the genetic disorder phenylketonuria, you should avoid its use. That's because you won't be able to metabolize phenylalanine, one of the two main components of aspartame.

Your expectations of weight-reducing aids should not be too high. Realize what they can and can't do. You shouldn't expect to take an OTC medication, continue your previous eating habits and level of activity —or inactivity—and expect the pounds to drop off.

The recommended products

The FDA advisory review panel on OTC Miscellaneous Internal Drug Products reviewed all such reducing aids in its report, "Weight-Control Drug Products for OTC Human Use." It found only two products—plus one combination—safe and effective: phenylpropanolamine hydrochloride (PPA) and benzocaine, an anesthetic. The combination product approved can contain PPA and 100 mg to 200 mg caffeine or caffeine citrate. The caffeine is approximately what you would get by drinking one cup of coffee. Although caffeine isn't responsible for weight loss, the FDA panel found it helps eliminate fatigue associated with attempts at losing weight.

Combination products containing vitamins and minerals were not approved. Nor were "starch blockers," also known as amylase inhibitors or blockers. Alpha amylase is an enzyme derived from the kidney bean. These starch blockers were popular a few years ago. They were purported to soak up all the starch from the food you ate so it could not be absorbed by the body and add calories and pounds. A great idea, but not effective.

The two approved active ingredients, PPA and benzocaine, work in the body in different ways to control weight. PPA's action is similar to amphetamines, prescription drugs used to reduce weight but dangerous because they can be addictive and easily abused. PPA does produce some side effects, including anxiety, excitement, headaches, and insomnia. Also, because PPA acts in the body by constricting capillaries, it speeds up the heart rate, and heartbeat irregularities may

Anorexia nervosa and bulimia

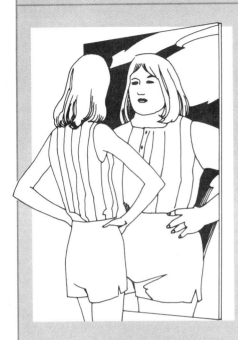

Anorexia nervosa and bulimia—also called bulimarexia—are eating disorders that people who diet should be aware of. Both are obsessions with food—the anorexic turns away from food, the bulimic toward it. These disorders usually begin in adolescence. Both require professional medical or psychological help. If you think you fit into either category, consult your doctor.

Anorexia nervosa is marked by an obsession—to the point of self-starvation—with thinness. The word *anorexia* means to "turn away from appetite." Often, however, even when a person looks emaciated to others, she will still perceive herself as being fat. Many doctors say women who become anorexics are rejecting feminity, because they diet to remove the curves associated with being female. Often anorexics are extremely intelligent people who feel they can't live up to others' expectations, but can exert control over themselves by what they eat—or don't eat. Many anorexics must be hospitalized when they become weak from not eating. They're usually fed intravenously to get their weight up to what's considered healthy.

Bulimia is different in that bulimics do eat, but they eat vast amounts of food and then purge it all by vomiting, fasting, or abusing laxatives. Most of this eating is done alone, in secret, and the food consumed is "junk food," high in calories and sugar. The women—and 90 to 95 percent of all bulimics are women—who fall into this category are perfectionists and overachievers; they're also low in self-esteem and dependent on others for approval. They believe that by being thin, they're being perfect. Jane Fonda, actress and exercise proponent, recently admitted to being caught up in the "binge/purge" cycle. Singer Karen Carpenter died of what is thought to have been an ipecac syrup overdose. Bulimics often abuse this drug to purge themselves after a binge. It's only within the past 10 years that bulimia has been recognized and treated. Most women suffered alone before then, unaware that anyone else had the same problem.

result. Overall, the FDA approved PPA in doses of 37.5 mg for regular doses and 75 mg for sustained-release products.

This decision was not without opposition. Some studies report that PPA does nothing long-term for obese patients and that people who use the product run the risk of raising their blood pressure. For that reason, the FDA requires a special warning for OTC medications containing PPA: "Do not exceed the recommended dosage. If nervousness, dizziness, or sleeplessness occur, stop the medication and consult your physician. If you are being treated for high blood pressure or depression, or have heart disease, diabetes, or thyroid disease, do not take this product except under the supervision of a physician."

Examples of products containing PPA are Coffee, Tea & A New Me, manufactured by Thompson Medical, and Dietac, manufactured by Menley & James. Combination products containing PPA and caffeine include Anorexin One-Span, made by SDA Pharmaceuticals, and Appress, made by North American. Both are timed-release capsules.

Benzocaine, an anesthetic, helps us lose weight by temporarily deadening our tastebuds. This works because many people eat to enjoy the taste of foods, particularly sweets. The FDA panel said that candy or chewing gum containing 3 mg to 15 mg of benzocaine is an effective way to lose weight. Slim-Line gum, made by Thompson Medical, is one OTC product that contains 6 mg benzocaine.

Quite a few active ingredients in weight-reducing aids were "conditionally approved" by the FDA panel. This means that they're safe for you to consume, but that their effectiveness in helping you lose weight remains to be proved.

These include alginic acid, carboxymethylcellulose sodium, carrageenan, chondrus, guar gum, karaya gum, methycellulose, psyllium, sea kelp, and xanthan gum. Many are made from plant cellulose, which absorbs water and produces bulky substances in the stomach, causing a full feeling.

Several other products were "summarily disapproved" by the FDA panel because neither their safety nor their effectiveness could be proved. They include sugars and sugar-substitutes such as fructose, dextrose, mannitol, sucrose, and saccharin; sodium; and other familiar products such as vitamins, wheat germ, and yeast.

19

Diagnostic tests

A free brochure
For a free brochure on
blood pressure from the
National Heart, Lung, and
Blood Institute, write to
The High Blood Pressure
Information Center, Na-
tional Institutes of Health,
Bethesda, MD 20215.

As far back as you can remember, you'll recall your parents taking your temperature with a thermometer. It was a way of telling whether you were sick enough to require a visit to your family doctor. The thermometer is a diagnostic tool you can use yourself to prevent unnecessary visits to the doctor.

From the simple thermometer, the home market for such diagnostic tools has boomed. In fact, according to a New York City research group, by 1990 consumers like you will spend more than $1 billion on diagnostic products you can take home.

The fastest-selling products are called test kits. These kits allow you to discover certain information about your body. The tests are similar to tests your doctor might perform. For example, if you suspect you're pregnant, you might want to use a test kit to find out. If the results are positive, you'll want to contact your doctor for a confirmation.

Besides pregnancy, you can buy test kits that monitor your glucose, which is important if you're a diabetic, or determine whether you have blood in your stool, a sign of colon or rectal cancer. You can also buy blood pressure machines, urine infection tests, and a venereal disease kit. Manufacturers are now developing test kits for anemia, breast cancer, cholesterol levels, hepatitis, kidney disease, and ulcers.

The FDA didn't examine diagnostic test kits when it was reviewing nonprescription drugs, because the kits don't contain any active drug ingredients used in or on the body. However, the agency can regulate the safety and effectiveness of these products under its Medical Device Amendment, passed by Congress in 1976.

Test kits are becoming more sophisticated. No longer do you have to follow complicated instructions and perform clumsy procedures or wait a long time before you get the results.

Blood pressure monitors

Blood pressure monitors you use at home come in several models.

Doctors recommend only patients with medical problems already diagnosed use these home machines; for example, if you're trying to monitor or control your blood pressure. About 25 percent of Americans suffer from high blood pressure. High blood pressure may run in the family, or it may be a result of pregnancy or use of oral contraceptives. It may also increase with age or weight.

If you buy a machine to use at home, take readings only twice a week.

Sometimes readings need to be done twice because the first might be off. However, a reading may vary as much as 10 to 15 mmHg within minutes.

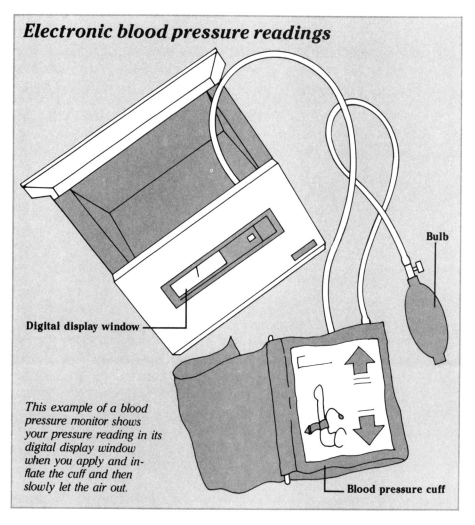

Electronic blood pressure readings

Bulb

Digital display window

This example of a blood pressure monitor shows your pressure reading in its digital display window when you apply and inflate the cuff and then slowly let the air out.

Blood pressure cuff

How to use thermometers

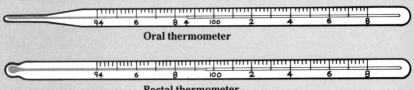

Oral thermometer

Rectal thermometer

You can use several different kinds of thermometers at home to check your temperature. The most familiar are the oral and rectal mercury thermometers, but today electronic oral and rectal thermometers and chemical-dot thermometers are available. Directions to use each are given below.

For mercury thermometers (both oral and rectal) four essential steps must be taken before inserting the thermometer.

• With your thumb and forefinger, grasp the thermometer at the end opposite the bulb.

• If the thermometer has been soaking in a disinfectant, rinse it in cold water.

• Then, quickly snap your wrist to shake down the mercury. If the thermometer isn't shaken down, the mercury will remain at the previous reading.

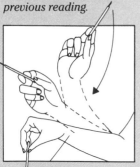

• Next, hold the thermometer at eye level in good light and rotate it slowly until the mercury line becomes visible. Check for a reading of 95° or less.

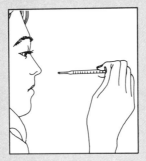

To take an oral temperature

• Place the bulb of the thermometer under your tongue, as far back as possible.

• Leave the thermometer in place for 4 to 5 minutes to register the correct temperature.

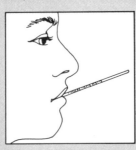

• Then, remove the thermometer and read it at eye level.

To take rectal temperature

In certain cases, taking a rectal temperature is preferred to taking an oral temperature—for instance, with children. Don't use an oral thermometer to take a rectal temperature. This procedure should not be attempted on oneself.

• Position the person on his or her side, with the top leg bent.

• Lubricate about ½ inch of the bulb of the thermometer for an infant, about 1½ inches for an adult.

• Next, lift the person's upper buttock, and gently insert the thermometer about ½ inch for an infant, 1½ inches for an adult.

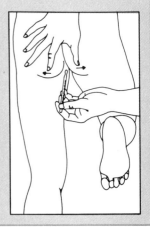

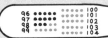

Disposable chemical-dot thermometer

• Hold the thermometer in place for 3 minutes.

• Carefully remove the thermometer and wipe it with a tissue.

• Read the thermometer at eye level, then shake down the mercury.

Electronic thermometers
To take an oral temperature with an electronic thermometer:

• Put the probe under your tongue, as far back as possible.

• Close your lips.

• Leave the probe in place until the maximum temperature appears on the digital display.

• After noting temperature, remove the probe from your mouth.

To take a rectal temperature with an electronic thermometer
If you need to take a person's temperature rectally with an electronic thermometer, you follow steps similar to those used with a mercury thermometer. Remember, you shouldn't take your own temperature rectally.

• Insert the rectal probe into a disposable probe cover.

• Position the person on his or her side, with the top leg bent.

• Lubricate the probe cover.

• Next, lift the patient's upper buttock, and gently insert the probe into the anus.

• Leave the probe in place until the maximum temperature appears on the digital display.

• After noting temperature, carefully remove the probe.

• Remove the probe cover and return to its holder.

To use a disposable chemical-dot thermometer
• Remove the thermometer from its protective case.

• Position the thermometer tip under your tongue, as far back as possible.

• Close your lips.

• Leave the thermometer in place for at least 45 seconds.

• Remove the thermometer and read the temperature as the last dye dot that has changed color.

• Discard the thermometer.

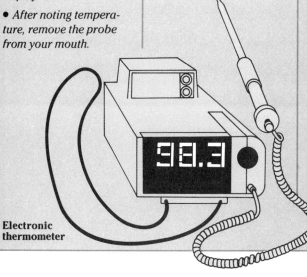

Electronic thermometer

Early pregnancy tests

Several companies have recently introduced early pregnancy tests that you can easily use in your home. The test is done in a small tube using your urine. Results are available in less than one hour. If the solution is one color, you're pregnant; if it's another, you're not. (Colors depend on the kit you buy.) Another benefit is that some kits are portable, so if you use the kit in the morning before you go out, you can take the test tube with you for results.

Tests such as these are called immunoassays because they detect in urine the hormone human chorionic gonadotropin, or HCG, which women produce when they're pregnant. These tests usually cost between $5 and $10 each and can't be reused. You may want to repeat the test a second time a week later for confirmation of the first finding.

Some doctors recommend waiting to use early pregnancy tests until two weeks after a missed period if a woman is regular or three weeks if she's not. Sometimes missed periods are caused by illness or stress. You should wait: your period may come. If it doesn't, the HCG hormone levels in your urine should then be high enough to make the home test accurate.

What's in a pregnancy test kit

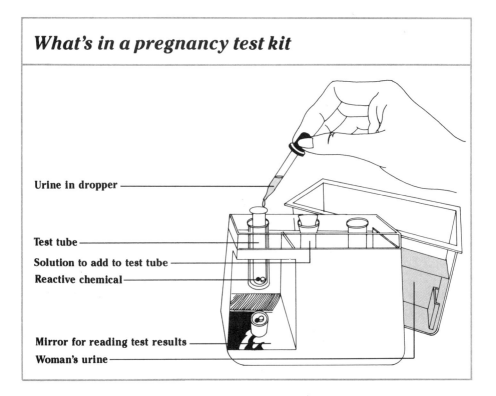

Urine in dropper

Test tube

Solution to add to test tube

Reactive chemical

Mirror for reading test results

Woman's urine

Colon and rectal cancer tests

Home test kits for colon cancer are also available. Colon cancer is the second most common form of cancer, but if you detect it early, treatment can be started. The American Cancer Society stresses that three-quarters of Americans discovered to have colon cancer every year could be cured if it were detected earlier.

The home tests for colon and rectal cancer—like those done at your doctor's office—look for blood hidden in stools. Two kits now being sold are Hemoccult (Menley & James) and Early Detector (Warner-Lambert). The latter involves patting the anal area with a specially prepared paper tissue after a bowel movement. A solution is then sprayed on the tissue. Color changes—in this case blue—indicate the presence of blood. Another test developed by Helena Laboratories eliminates the need for stool samples. Instead a ColoScreen Self-Test (CS-T™) pretreated pad is dropped into the toilet after a bowel movement. A red color indicates the presence of blood. The colorectal tests cost between $5 and $10.

Colon and rectal tests

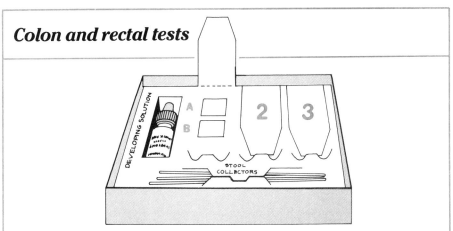

Stool test kits are available for use at home to check for potential problems in the lower intestinal tract. These tests are designed to detect blood in the stool. Blood in the stool could be caused by a number of conditions. See your doctor if your test is positive.

Stool tests use special paper coated in a substance that's sensitive to blood. When you add a small stool sample that has blood in it, the paper turns a color to indicate the presence of blood.

You'll have to follow a special diet before you use one of these kits. Read the directions for use 3 to 5 days before you plan to use the test, because the diet must be followed for several days before the test is done.

Remember, this test can't replace a rectal examination by your doctor.

The American Cancer Society worries that you might not recognize the blood when you see it. Also, presence of blood can indicate other conditions, such as ulcers, colitis, polyps that are not cancerous, or even hemorrhoids. If you do suspect the presence of blood after using one of the test kits, contact your doctor for a retest. If colon cancer runs in your family or you're over 40, you should be tested by a doctor once a year anyway.

Accuracy of home test kits

One problem with any home kit is its accuracy. As technology develops, these products will become more and more sensitive. But any test based on body wastes, such as urine or stools, may not be accurate all the time, even when performed in a doctor's office. For example, an early pregnancy test kit may tell you're not pregnant when you are. This is called a "false negative." There are also "false positives": the kit tells you you're pregnant when you're not.

Check the instructions in home kits carefully to determine what the percentage rate of false negatives and false positives is. For example, a false negative rate of 11.2 percent indicates that the test will miss what it's looking for 11.2 percent of the time.

Any questions you have about your health can be best answered by your doctor. Home test kits may save some visits, but you shouldn't rely on them completely.

20

Poisoning emergencies

Lifesaving information
Your telephone book lists the number of the poison control center near you. Look it up now and record it on or near your telephone.

Poison control centers
Poison control centers are usually affiliated with a hospital and staffed by specialists in toxicology. If you call a poison control center with a problem, you'll need to describe what happened, and tell if you know what the poison or drug was—in cases of suspected overdose. Then they'll tell you what to do.

Most poison control centers use sophisticated, computerized data banks that instantly search out the problem and the correct procedure. You'll help speed the information gathering if you have the container the poison or drug came in. That way, you can name the particular brand, drug, or ingredient.

Some cases of accidental overdoses and poisoning emergencies—such as a child swallowing a handful of aspirin tablets—call for induced vomiting. You should always keep a bottle of ipecac syrup on hand to promote vomiting.

Before giving a poisoning victim ipecac syrup, you should call a poison control center. In some cases, vomiting may not be necessary, and in some cases it can be dangerous (for example, if the victim has swallowed a corrosive, or burning, substance or if the victim is having convulsions).

Ipecac syrup

If advised to do so by the poison control center, give the victim ipecac syrup. If the victim doesn't vomit within 20 to 30 minutes, repeat the entire procedure. If the victim still doesn't vomit, contact the poison control center for further advice.

Age	Dosage	Water
Small child	1 to 2 Teaspoons	1/2 to 1 glass
Adult or older child	1 Tablespoon	2 glasses

21 Of special interest to women

Douching daily?
The FDA panel found no reason women can't douche daily if they want to, but it recommended that such products be used only as anti-irritants and cleansers.

It seems almost natural that obsession with body odor should extend to the genitals. By the early 1970s, more than 30 different brands of "feminine hygiene sprays" were on the market. However, many caused allergic reactions. Like many other parts of the body, the vagina is capable of keeping itself clean. Therefore, the best remedy remains soap and water and careful drying of the area. If you must use a spray, check the ingredients on the label for any you may be allergic to. Hold the spray nozzle about 8 inches away for best results.

Douches

Douching is a way of cleaning out, or irrigating, the vagina. The FDA panel found no reason women can't douche daily if they want to, but it recommended that such products be used only as anti-irritants and cleansers. Some women like to douche after intercourse to feel clean. However, douching does not prevent pregnancy. Others may wish to cleanse their vaginas after menstruating to wash out remaining particles of blood or mucus. You shouldn't douche if you're pregnant.

The FDA panel found calcium propionate, sodium propionate, and potassium sorbate (Summer's Eve Medicated Disposable Douche, Fleet) safe and effective anti-irritants. No acidifiers or alkalizers—including commonly used vinegar—were found effective, but they're safe.

Safe and effective detergent cleansers include products with the ingredients docusate sodium and sodium lauryl sulfate, and nonoxynol-9 and octoxynol 9. The last two are both found in spermicides.

Vaginitis and yeast infections

Vaginitis and yeast infections are problems most women can treat themselves. Vaginitis can be either the upsetting of natural microorganisms that live in the vagina or an attack from the outside. It's marked by itching, burning, odor, and irritation of the genital area. Aggravations can include tight clothing, wet bathing suits, hot and humid weather, deodorant perfumes, too much douching, poor vaginal hygiene, or use of diaphragms and IUDs (intrauterine device).

The yeasts are *Candida albicans,* naturally present in the vagina. Sometimes infections may not be caused by these yeasts, but more often than not they are. A close runner-up is "tric," another form of vaginitis caused by *Trichomonas vaginalis.* Because both occur frequently, and women are capable of recognizing them, the FDA panel was in favor of reclassifying two prescription drug ingredients to OTC status. They're haloprogin and miconazole nitrate; neither has been reclassified yet. The hydrocortisones, recommended as topicals for itching skin, can be used outside the vagina but not inside.

Menstrual problems

Most women menstruate regularly approximately every month from about the time they're 11 until they're 55. Each month, certain symptoms accompany menstruation, including headaches, a swollen, bloated feeling, nausea, cramps, and grouchiness. The market for "menstrual distress preparations" is big.

Three ingredients are sold or promoted as diuretics for the premenstrual swelling and bloated feeling. They are ammonium chloride, caffeine, and pamabron. Diuretics, or water pills, should only be used premenstrually, the FDA panel stresses. If you're taking them for any other reason, see your doctor immediately.

Toxic shock syndrome

When you menstruate, it really doesn't matter whether you choose a pad or a tampon to contain the menstrual flow. Most women use what their mothers did or what they've found most comfortable from experimenting with different products. However, you should be aware of toxic shock syndrome, or TSS, first reported in 1978. It was originally linked to Rely Tampons, manufactured by Procter & Gamble. The company immediately recalled this product after reports of deaths from TSS. The disease is marked by a high fever, vomiting, diarrhea, a rash followed by peeling of the skin, and a drop in blood pressure so rapid you may go into shock.

TSS isn't caused by tampon use, however, and even men and children can get it. It's caused by the common bacterium Staphylococcus aureus. Since 1978, scientists have found that the critical issues are use of a tampon rather than a pad and the material used in the tampon. Polyester tampons are preferred over natural fibers.

To be on the safe side, use a pad or minipad, which fits in the underwear. If you must use a tampon, choose one with the least amount of absorbency you can use comfortably. Change tampons frequently. You can also combine use of a tampon during the day and a minipad at night. Also, if you use a diaphragm, don't leave it in longer than recommended by your doctor.

Index